Anxiety Workbook for Men

Anxiety Workbook

FOR MEN

Evidence-Based Exercises to Manage Anxiety, Depression, and Worry

SIMON G. NIBLOCK, MA, LMFT

ROCKRIDGE
PRESS

Interior and Cover Designer: Sean Doyle
Art Producer: Tom Hood
Editors: Meera Pal and Samantha Holland
Production Editor: Emily Sheehan
Production Manager: Michael Kay

Cover and interior illustration courtesy of West Wind Creative/Creative Market; Author photograph courtesy of Paige Casey.

ISBN: Print 978-1-64876-694-7 | eBook 978-1-64876-191-1
R0

*I dedicate this book to my dad, Tom.
The bloke who taught me to paddle hard
toward the oncoming wave and to savor the
cold spray rising from the bow.*

Contents

Introduction viii

How to Use This Book x

CHAPTER 1:
Deciphering Anxiety
1

CHAPTER 2:
Get Familiar with Your Anxiety
23

CHAPTER 3:
Managing Your Anxiety
41

CHAPTER 4:
Recognize & Challenge
Negative Thinking
51

CHAPTER 5:
Conquering Fear of the Unknown
71

CHAPTER 6:
Handling Difficult Emotions
87

CHAPTER 7:
Jumping Through Hurdles
101

CHAPTER 8:
In Your Body
125

CHAPTER 9:
Meet Your Fears Head-On
137

CHAPTER 10:
Find Your Calm
151

CHAPTER 11:
Choose Your Path
165

Resources 173

References 175

Index 182

Introduction

The gentleman who sat opposite me in my office, dressed in a rumpled suit, easily could have been placed in any city you can picture—London, New York, Sydney, Singapore, Los Angeles. The problem he was seeking professional help with knows no boundaries and is a growing global problem. The problem: anxiety.

The man explained, "I might look good on paper, but my life is miserable. I'm racked by this constant angst, this fear of making the wrong decisions, fear of being caught out. I'm spending most of my time and mental energy just trying to figure out what's wrong—and I have no idea what to do. I'm drinking more than ever before, and I'm at my wits' end."

As a licensed marriage and family therapist specializing in mental and relationship therapy for men for the past decade, I find that this conversation is all too familiar. Among the biggest issues facing the men who find the courage to pick up the phone or walk into my office is the pervasive and intrusive nature of anxiety.

I'm not talking about the garden-variety anxiety you might experience before an exam or a job interview. I'm describing something far more intrusive and impactful. It's the growing prevalence of fear, uncertainty, and doubt—and how it shapes and distorts men's thoughts, emotions, and behaviors. More important, it's how men find themselves stuck in its vicious cycle, until they implode, explode, or find a solution.

I first recognized the growing creature of anxiety when I drank from the firehose of the corporate world for almost 25 years. The stories that my male colleagues would share about their state of mind, and the colorful ways they found to cope, were eye-opening. The pressure, the uncertainty, and the excessiveness of it all frequently took a toll.

The trend was blatantly obvious and disturbing. This insight prompted me to seek an alternative career, providing professional support and guidance for men whose well-being had been drastically compromised by anxiety and other culprits.

Thousands of clinical conversations later, I recognize that regardless of upbringing, socioeconomic status, race, ethnicity, culture, or identity, men struggle with anxiety in very concerning ways. As demands and expectations evolve in our fast-paced contemporary life, men's burden of anxiety is on the rise. It's no surprise that they, more than ever, are desperate to find practical and enduring ways to improve the quality of their lives.

Eventually, the gentleman who came to me seeking help found calm and clarity in his life. The work that he bravely undertook wasn't always easy. Yet he was able to disrupt the cycle of anxiety that had entrapped him. The day came when he departed my office a very different person. Here was a man who wasn't afraid of the fears that he—like many men—had constructed in his own mind. The gates of his cage had been opened, and he stepped through. His departing words to me were that he felt free for the first time and that he was genuinely optimistic about his life ahead.

This true story highlights the arrival and departure of one of my clients. But the time in between is where the story really happened. He, like many other men who came seeking help with their anxiety, ventured on this journey in hopes of a better life. Working through anxiety is truly a journey, one that involves education, increased awareness, introspection, and courage. To work through it requires an understanding of how men are uniquely affected by anxiety and a willingness to open up to the possibility of learning more about ourselves. The reward for this work is a life filled with potential, freedom from the strictures of emotional barriers, and knowledge to disarm anxiety should it arise again.

If this journey speaks to you, I'm very glad you're here.

How to Use This Book

Welcome! Chances are, if you've picked up this workbook, you're feeling a disconnect from the life you envision for yourself, caused by the invasive experience of anxiety.

Maybe you sought out this book. Or maybe someone recommended it to you because they are worried that you're struggling. There's no shame in that at all. Sometimes we gentlemen need a bit of encouragement to get things going.

This workbook was created with several essential things in mind. Not all men want to seek professional support. This workbook serves to respect and uphold their autonomy and self-agency. Equally, there are many men, and individuals who identify as men, who have limited access to professional support due to the high cost or lack of availability of suitable resources. This workbook aims to circumvent these barriers by offering a cost-effective, self-guided resource that contains many of the practical tools used in contemporary therapy.

This workbook is a customizable resource that works toward increasing your knowledge of the cause and effect of anxiety, while introducing you to a range of practical tips, tools, and tactics that you can adapt according to your needs and at your own pace.

This workbook does not strive to eliminate anxiety. That is not humanly possible. Anxiety plays a purposeful role in our life, as you're about to discover. Rather, it's the intrusive and debilitating anxiety that we're targeting here.

The purpose of this book is to help you step back from your anxiety experience to explore and challenge it from an objective and informed perspective. This is significant, because when you are caught in the cycle of anxiety, it feels brutally personal. This book strives to help you understand and alleviate the impact and burden that anxiety has inflicted.

It's essential to convey that this workbook is not a substitute for professional support, such as psychotherapy or medical guidance. If you recognize that you need professional help, seek assistance from a licensed mental health provider. See the Resources section (page 173) for some suggestions.

Here's what you can expect as you guide yourself through this workbook:

In chapter 1, you'll learn key concepts surrounding what anxiety is, what causes it to evolve, and which techniques are most successful in overcoming it. Chapter 2 is aimed at helping you shine a light on the causes and symptoms of your anxiety, including your unique triggers. Chapter 3 introduces cognitive behavioral therapy (CBT) and techniques such as mindfulness and meditation practices, acceptance and commitment therapy

(ACT), and clinical hypnotherapy. And in chapter 4, we'll explore the negative thinking cycle and how it influences how we interpret and respond to ambiguous situations.

Chapter 5 discusses fear of the unknown and why uncertainty can be difficult to tolerate. Chapter 6 will teach you how to manage difficult or intrusive emotions, rather than avoiding situations that evoke pain or fear. In both chapters, you'll be introduced to a range of tools and tactics that can help you deal with these issues. And in chapter 7, we'll discuss hurdles that most men learn to overcome as they tackle anxiety, including worrying, procrastination, and other forms of avoidance.

Chapter 8 discusses the relationship between anxiety and the body, including the concept of the mind-body connection, and you'll see how self-awareness can help reduce and mitigate the impact of anxiety. In chapter 9, you'll learn how exposure therapy can help effectively engage your fears. And in chapter 10, we'll explore how to foster calm through self-care practices, including sleep, nourishment, exercise, and relaxation techniques.

In the final chapter, you're invited to bring together everything you've learned throughout the workbook to develop a personalized practice plan that you can incorporate into your everyday life.

However, before we kick things off, I would like to offer you this thought: You are not your anxiety. You are not broken, dysfunctional, or faulty. You are a reservoir of untapped potential, and it's time to explore what that potential could be. Let's begin!

CHAPTER 1

Deciphering Anxiety

Before embarking on any new pursuit, it's best to get a lay of the land. In this first chapter, you'll be introduced to a number of key concepts aimed at helping you understand what anxiety actually is, what causes it to develop, and which techniques are most successful at mitigating it.

We'll examine the unique and often creative ways men respond to and manage anxiety, as well as how anxiety impacts men physically, cognitively, emotionally, and behaviorally. We'll also look at various contributing causes, such as environment and genetics.

Ready to kick things off? Let's go.

Anxiety and Men

Anxiety is a universal yet highly subjective personal experience. Anxiety impacts people regardless of their age, gender, and cultural or socioeconomic background. While researchers acknowledge that the causes of anxiety may differ for men and women, how they experience physical and psychological symptoms is relatively the same.

Research also highlights that while a greater number of women report experiencing anxiety, men are less likely to seek professional help. According to the National Survey on Drug Use and Health, women are almost twice as likely to utilize mental health services as men (17.7 percent of women versus 9.5 percent of men).

The report also highlighted that men are less likely than women to use outpatient mental health services and less likely to use prescription medication for mental health issues. The reasoning is twofold: First, men are not typically well versed in recognizing the signs of anxiety. Second, many men do not seek help because they think sharing or disclosing their experience is not considered masculine behavior. This lack of knowledge and reluctance to "go public" with a problem places men in a precarious bind.

When they do seek help, they often downplay or misrepresent their symptoms, resulting in misdiagnosis and ineffective treatment outcomes. This is because men respond to and express anxiety in very different ways than women. Men are often inclined to present anxiety in "secondary" emotional, physical, or behavioral ways. In other words, anxiety often sits beneath some other form of presentation; for example, expressing anger or aggression (a secondary emotion) rather than conveying fear or apprehension (a primary emotion). This is because anger is, hypocritically, a more socially accepted form of emotional expression for men than for women.

In men, anxiety may express itself in secondary emotional or physical forms such as:

- Anger
- Irritability or "being on edge"
- Restlessness
- Depressed mood
- Fatigue and/or burnout
- Difficulty concentrating or being present
- Sexual health issues (such as erectile dysfunction)

Men are also more inclined to adopt compensatory behaviors that serve as coping strategies for their anxiety, such as:

- Antisocial behavior or withdrawing
- Risky behaviors or activities
- Addictive behaviors (such as pornography or gaming)
- Substance abuse

These secondary and compensatory behaviors are often what lead men to seek help, either through their own volition or at the urging of a partner or colleague. So what's behind the fact that men are less likely to seek help for anxiety? Let's explore more deeply some of the very real reasons this happens.

Insecurities

There are many reasons men are reluctant to seek professional help for their anxiety (or any other mental health issue), including that they often struggle to identify the underlying issue and find it difficult to verbalize what's going on.

Here's what else: Many men are coached from a very young age that emotional expression or vulnerability is a weakness. This hypermasculine narrative is cultivated by conventional social and cultural systems such as education, sports, media institutions, and even family. These systems have made it very challenging for some men to accept that they can't do everything on their own. The expectation to be overly independent, strong, and self-reliant can cause discomfort and shame for a man who finds himself in a struggle he can't resolve alone, leading him to feel like a failure. In reality, he simply lacks the knowledge and resources required to identify and solve his problem.

Further adding to men's insecurities is the fact that many men are simply not accustomed to feeling like it's okay to open up to anyone about their struggles the way women do. Their network is also typically much smaller.

Social Stigmas/Norms

Society also plays a role in the stigma around men and mental health. According to the World Health Organization, the "cultural stigma surrounding mental health is one of the chief obstacles to people admitting they are struggling and seeking help, and this stigmatization is particularly pronounced in men."

It's culturally acceptable to enlist the help of experts in many fields—men turn to physical trainers for their physique, mechanics for their automobiles, and financial advisers for their money management. While it makes sense to call upon a mental health professional when that kind of support is needed, cultural norms condition men to reject help in favor of remaining emotionally in control and self-reliant.

Finding adequate help can also be problematic due to the lack of available mental health services focused on the needs of men, particularly men belonging to minority groups. Part of the problem is that many forms of mental health support run in direct opposition to how some men prefer to receive support. For example, talk therapy emphasizes the significance of sharing and experiencing emotions, something that a lot of men feel uncomfortable doing. Men also prefer mental health support to be solution- or action-oriented. For many men, the idea of engaging in an unstructured, continuous conversation doesn't align with their vision of getting better.

By the time a man does make it into a therapist's office, he's typically endured a lot of suffering and loss. This suffering and loss impacts the people around him—his partner, children, parents, and colleagues. During such vulnerable times, it's important to remember that asking for help is not a weakness; conversely, it's a sign of strength and courage.

Judgment-Free Zone

For some men, considering support for anxiety may feel like a daunting, even impossible task. The thought of reaching out evokes ambiguous thoughts and uncomfortable emotions. It's important to know that you're not alone. These thoughts are universal and valid.

Please take a moment to reflect on the possible reasons it's been challenging to seek help. Remember, this is a judgment-free zone. Answering the following questions openly and honestly goes a long way in helping you seek the change you envision for yourself. Write your answers in the lines provided.

- What possible reasons may have prevented you from seeking help with anxiety?

  ....

  ....

  ....

- What event(s) or occurence(s) prompted you to seek a solution now?

  ....

  ....

  ....

- If you were successful in addressing anxiety, how would you envision your life? What would be different?

....

....

....

- How do you hope this workbook will serve you in achieving this vision?

....

....

....

How Anxiety Can Show Up Differently for Men

Anxiety affects all individuals, regardless of gender identity, largely in the same way. However, the difference is in the way that those who identify as men or as masculine manage, process, and express their anxiety.

While women are traditionally nurtured with the notion that it's acceptable to show emotions, weakness, or vulnerability, men are typically not. Men are often socialized from a young age to suppress their emotions. Suppression refers to the internal prohibition of emotions. Emotional suppression can lead men to dissociate from what they feel. As a result, it can lead to dysfunctional or avoidant behaviors to keep uncomfortable or unfamiliar emotions at bay.

In individuals with an anxiety-related disorder, accompanying issues (also referred to as *comorbid disorders*) are more common among men. Studies show that men's anxiety is commonly accompanied by an additional issue such as substance abuse, disruptive impulse control, or antisocial behavior.

Men develop these alternative ways of expressing themselves, but they will struggle to recognize that these behaviors are actually related to anxiety. This is because men often attempt to resolve anxiety using methods that are consistent with masculine constructs such as independence, strength, courage, and assertiveness.

There is nothing wrong with any of these masculine constructs—that is, until they are paradoxically used to avoid something that could be harmful. An example of this might be knowing that you're sick and refusing to go to the doctor because you think that asking for help shows weakness.

To avoid anxiety, men will frequently divert their attention to various activities or pursuits, including work, education, leisure, watching pornography, and exercise. Others seek thrilling or risky experiences that place their safety and well-being in jeopardy.

Gents, don't neglect your health because you believe you're supposed to "tough it out." Be the most formidable advocate for your own state of mind and well-being.

Let's look at some of the more common ways men typically express anxiety.

Substance Abuse

Men often turn to substances such as alcohol or drugs to help numb their emotions or help them cope with the underlying experience of anxiety, even if the anxiety is not immediately apparent to them.

Substance abuse includes the persistent and harmful use of an ingredient or substance, either legal (such as alcohol, nicotine, or prescription medication) or illegal (such as heroin, cocaine, or methamphetamines), which can lead to significant long-term difficulties. While men may turn to these substances for temporary relief, the use of these substances can actually prolong symptoms of anxiety and, in many cases, exacerbate its effects and consequences.

Anger

One of the most predominant behavioral expressions of anxiety for men is anger. Like each of our respective emotions, anger surfaces when we face a perceived or actual threat to our well-being, which includes our sense of self and our view of fairness or morality. Anger is experienced in a variety of states and intensities, ranging from simple annoyance to frustration, exasperation, argumentativeness, bitterness, vengefulness, and fury.

Because of early-learned masculine constructs, anger is considered a socially accepted method for men to manage emotions such as fear and discomfort. For some, anger creates the perception of being in control, particularly when they feel helpless or hopeless, which evokes deep emotions such as vulnerability or fear.

Men who experience anger often report intense emotional flooding, accompanied by other physical symptoms such as an increased heartbeat, sweating, flushing (sudden reddening of the face, neck, or upper chest due to increased blood flow), and the sensation that their anger seems difficult to control or regulate. This becomes an issue when anger is frequent or expressed through verbal outbursts and/or physical aggression or violence.

Irritability

Irritability is considered a relative to anger. It is a frequent component of a number of mental health disorders and is particularly associated with generalized anxiety. With irritability, even minor things can evoke annoyance and agitation. When irritation persists over a prolonged period, the tension can lead to a greater sensitivity to stressful situations.

Men often report experiencing the physical symptoms of irritability as increased sensations of heat, tension, or restlessness, as well as a change in mental processes, often accompanied by an inability to cope or concentrate. Those close to men who struggle with persistent irritability will often describe these men as being grouchy, impatient, agitated, or argumentative.

Depression

Depression is a common mood disorder characterized by a persistently depressed mood or loss of interest in activities, causing significant impairment in daily life. Also referred to as *major depressive disorder* or *clinical depression*, it affects how someone thinks, feels, and behaves and can lead to various emotional and physical problems.

Depression is usually accompanied by behavioral and physical symptoms, which may include changes in sleeping habits, appetite and weight, energy level, concentration, daily behavior, or self-esteem.

While the underlying cause of depression is still unknown, some consider anxiety and depression to be more closely related than is often medically recognized. It's easy to see how anxiety, left untreated, can evolve into a depressed state or full-blown depression.

If you can relate, know that there is always hope. You don't have to give in to anxiety and depression—there are surefire ways to address them both. By working through this book, you can learn to manage your anxiety to alleviate depression.

Developing Awareness

Developing an awareness of your own anxiety experience is a vital first step toward finding calmness and clarity. By completing this workbook, you can quickly become a master of this highly important skill.

Take a moment to reflect on your experience using the following questions.

- What happens to me physically when I experience anxiety?

- What happens to me emotionally when I experience anxiety?

- What do I find myself doing (my actions) or wanting to do when I experience anxiety?

- What thoughts do I have when I experience anxiety?

What Is Anxiety?

Anxiety is one of the most universal experiences of our modern world and an anticipated part of life. We can experience it when we're going for a job interview, giving a presentation, making an important decision, or having a sensitive conversation with a loved one. However, for some, the fear and dread commonly experienced with anxiety are more dominant, even debilitating at times.

The *Diagnostic and Statistical Manual of Mental Health Disorders*, Fifth Edition, or DSM-5, introduces the umbrella term of "anxiety disorders," which explains a range of mental health issues with similar fear- and anxiety-related features and frequently the same negative behavioral consequences. For many with these disorders, fear is the primary response to an actual or sensed threat. On the other hand, anxiety is primarily the anticipation of a future threat that does not yet exist. (We'll get more into this later on.)

While occasional or situational fear and/or anxiety are everyday experiences in life, it can be disabling for many who suffer from an anxiety disorder. Persistent anxiety can lead to adverse consequences, impacting our ability to think, feel, and act and generally limiting our ability to flourish.

Each individual's anxiety experience is unique, with various symptoms that appear interwoven. The following is an example of how anxiety can present itself. (Please note that identifying information in all anecdotes has been changed to protect confidentiality.)

> *Brian is a high-tech sales professional who typically enjoys his job and the demands and pressures that come with it. Over the past six months, Brian has noticed some unusual physical symptoms when interacting with his colleagues and engaging in routine work tasks. His chest starts to tighten, and his heart flutters. His hands feel clammy, and he struggles to remain in control and concentrate. While he attributes these physical symptoms to the pressures of the job, he has begun to worry about his ability to do his job effectively. Brian is usually a highly social person, but he has recently declined a number of opportunities to have drinks with his colleagues after work, preferring to leave early.*

Anxiety and Your Body

People are relatively in tune with their bodies and the physical symptoms of anxiety, even if they don't specifically recognize that they are struggling with a particular anxiety disorder. The brain and body are intricately connected in that they both respond to the perception of danger.

Anxiety activates the autonomic nervous system, commonly described as the body's "fight or flight" response. Its role is facilitated by two components: the sympathetic nervous system and the parasympathetic nervous system.

Generally, the sympathetic division does most of the work during moments of high anxiety in that it prepares the body for stressful or emergency situations. Immediate physiological consequences include hyperventilation (rapid breathing, shortness of breath, sweating, cold/clammy hands, paling or flushing) and cardiovascular system response (pounding heart or increased heart rate, chest pain, and increased blood pressure).

Prolonged anxiety can have long-term physical consequences, such as impaired immune function (loss of energy, headaches, insomnia, muscle pain) and digestive function (nausea or digestive trouble, diarrhea, and irritable bowel syndrome).

Anxiety and Your Brain

Just as there is a lot of action in the body when anxiety kicks in, there is also a lot of activity in the brain. The brain activates an arousal system during adversity. This is the stress response, which includes a series of nervous system arousals in preparation for danger—we are essentially being primed to evade or combat a particular situation or stimuli.

Traditionally, it was thought that the central part of the brain that triggered this response, and therefore controlled fear and anxiety, was the amygdala. The amygdala's role is the processing of emotions such as fear, anger, and pleasure. However, researchers now suspect that anxiety results from constant chatter among several different brain regions, described as a "fear network." This adds to the complexity of how we look at the brain to determine how best to treat anxiety.

When Anxiety Gets in the Way

Many men tend to seek professional help when they recognize that the things they desire fail to come to fruition.

It is natural for anyone to want to flourish or prosper. We have an innate tendency to move toward what we are meant to become—to pursue our fullest potential. In physiological terms, this state is called "self-actualization."

The concept of self-actualization represents a notion derived from humanistic psychological theory and from Abraham Maslow, creator of the theory. According to Maslow, self-actualization represents an individual's growth toward fulfillment of the highest needs—particularly the need for meaning in life.

Anxiety can drastically restrict an individual's willingness and ability to seek improvements in many life domains, including relationships, vocation and career, and personal performance. Quality of life is the most significant way in which an anxiety disorder can affect you. To have an anxiety disorder is to live in fear, and often fear of nothing in particular, and life is too short to be afraid of our own shadows. But thankfully, there is much we can do to work through anxiety and reclaim our place as the driver of our success, as you'll learn in upcoming chapters.

In Case of Emergency

Navigating a mental health crisis can be daunting. If you are experiencing a mental health emergency, seek professional help immediately. Call 911 or visit your nearest emergency room for immediate assistance. If you are experiencing suicidal thoughts or are concerned about self-harm, call the National Suicide Prevention Lifeline at 1 (800) 273-8255 or visit their website at SuicidePreventionLifeline.org (United States only).

There are also other resources. If you have insurance, call the behavioral health number on the back of your health insurance card. You can inquire whether your employer offers an Employee Assistance Program (EAP). Alternately, call a local counseling office and schedule an urgent appointment.

Gentlemen, there is no shame in seeking help. You are not alone.

Anxiety Is Equal Opportunity

While the human experience is vast in its diversity, there are some experiences shared by all. Anxiety happens to be one of them. But it isn't all bad—anxiety serves an important function, as it helps alert us to danger or prepare us for potentially stressful situations. It also assists us with learning development and our ability to adapt, plan for the future, and meet the challenges of day-to-day life. Under ordinary circumstances, anxiety is a natural performance-enhancing behavior that keeps us on our toes when we need it most. However, the beneficial effects of anxiety are limited to those who experience only moderate anxiety. When anxiety is more severe, it actually leads to deterioration in performance. Heightened and prolonged anxiety can develop into an illness or disorder.

What makes understanding anxiety a bit complicated is that even when faced with the exact same stressors, some people experience debilitating anxiety while others are able to successfully mitigate the effects. Multiple models attempt to explain why some seem more prone to anxiety than others, using what is known about biological and environmental factors. We'll explore these factors here.

Environmental Factors

Throughout life, just about everyone deals with environmental stressors, from losing a job or a loved one to experiencing illness, injury, or trauma. Adverse situations like these are the main source of anxiety for most men.

The sudden or unexpected nature of some environmental stressors can evoke tremendous stress and uncertainty about the future. The saying "waiting for the other shoe to drop" is a good way of describing what it feels like when you're reeling from one adverse event and anxious that another may occur. Environmental stressors can indeed trigger the development of an anxiety disorder.

There are additional environmental factors, including adverse childhood experiences (ACEs). An adverse childhood experience can include violence, abuse, or neglect, having a family member attempt or die by suicide, substance abuse, mental health problems, as well as family instability, separation, or incarceration. The greater the number of adverse experiences, the greater the risk for mental health disorders in life. According to research, about 61 percent of adults surveyed reported that they had experienced at least one ACE, and nearly one in six reported they had experienced four or more ACEs.

Genetic Factors

Environmental factors may create stressful situations, but genetics plays a role in how well we are able to adapt to those situations. Researchers have found that genetic vulnerability, combined with specific environmental stressors, can trigger symptoms of a mental health disorder. In other words, who you are on a genetic level can play a role in how well you cope with what happens to you on an emotional level.

As with many other health conditions, a person can be genetically predisposed to developing specific symptoms, such as anxiety. Science has yet to establish a firm understanding of how genes influence our ability to develop a mental disorder. So far, we understand that you may be more likely to develop anxiety if genetic markers associated with anxiety are passed on from your parents. For example, generalized anxiety disorder is a heritable condition with a moderate genetic risk of up to 30 percent. This implies that people who have family members with anxiety are more likely to experience anxiety themselves.

Anxiety vs. Fear

There is a broad debate about the intersection of anxiety and fear, but they are two very different states. Fear is a primary emotion that is present-focused, usually rational, and a reaction to a specific, observable danger. Anxiety is considered future-oriented and is a generalized response to an unknown threat or internal conflict. Let's dive into them in more detail.

Fear is an important survival emotion. It serves to protect by automatically kicking in all the mental, physical, and behavioral traits needed when faced with potential danger. It's not uncommon to experience surprise immediately before a fear response is activated. All of this happens within milliseconds. Fear is a universal response to a threat to our emotional or physical well-being that is real, present, and imminent.

At times, our brains cannot distinguish between an actual and imagined threat—such as a real tiger that's about to pounce and an imaginary one, which I often refer to as a "paper tiger." A paper tiger is best described as a thing, person, or situation that appears to be powerful or threatening but is actually a flimsy façade you can overcome. Luckily, we don't have too many real tigers casually wandering about these days.

Anxiety is a much more prolonged, complex emotional state often triggered by an initial fear. It's a state of apprehension and physical arousal where we believe we can't control or predict potentially adverse future events. We become anxious about imagined future adverse events or catastrophes.

Fear can evolve into anxiety if uncertainty or discomfort are experienced persistently without valid justification. Anxiety can quickly become irrational because it's untethered from real events—the imagination takes over, and humans can be very imaginative. At the heart of this process is a sense of uncontrol, mainly focused on possible future threats or danger. The brain is incredibly untamed when it's on imagination overload.

Forms of Anxiety

Anxiety is the chameleon of mental health disorders. While anxiety is used to describe the general state that many individuals experience, it can present itself in many forms.

The characteristics of anxiety can include:

- Exaggerated intensity
- Persistence
- Daily life interference
- Panic
- Generalization
- Catastrophic thinking
- Avoidance or withdrawal
- Loss of safety
- Agitation

Although anxiety is a highly universal disorder, not everyone experiences it in the same way, nor will everyone have all of these symptoms. On an individual level, anxiety can vary significantly in its intensity, frequency, and symptoms. Symptoms can be highly observable or shrewdly obscured.

According to the DSM-5, several distinct anxiety-related disorders fall under the general classification of anxiety. These include generalized anxiety, social anxiety, phobias, panic attacks, and worry. We'll cover these disorders in more detail soon.

It's important not to fall into the trap of diagnosing ourselves. The descriptions of the anxiety-related disorders are simply guidelines based on generalized, observable, and universal descriptions of particular symptoms. Speak with your doctor if you are experiencing any of the symptoms outlined in this section.

As complex and unique as we are as individuals, so are the emotional challenges that we experience. No single diagnostic criteria will correspond precisely to you as a person. This is important to remember as you navigate your own experience of anxiety.

Generalized Anxiety

Generalized anxiety disorder (GAD) is the most commonly experienced anxiety-related disorder. It's defined by excessive worry or repeated thinking about potential future events that are typically out of proportion to the actual likelihood or impact of the anticipated event.

Individuals report difficulty in stopping their worrying and often note that worrying about one topic leads to worrying about another. This "meta-worry" can dominate a person's thinking so much that it interferes with daily functioning—mainly social, occupational, or other personal functioning areas.

Symptoms of GAD also include restlessness, feeling keyed up or on edge, fatigue, having difficulty concentrating or "going blank," irritability, muscle tension, and disturbed sleep.

GAD must typically be experienced for at least six months to be identified as a disorder.

Social Anxiety

The essential feature of social anxiety disorder (SAD) is a marked or intense hypersensitivity to real or imaginary threats in social situations that occurs for longer than six months.

Individuals typically experience fear associated with the prospect of being scrutinized or judged as anxious, weak, crazy, stupid, dull, intimidating, dirty, or unlikable. As a result, some people fear offending others or being rejected. Individuals who experience social anxiety typically overestimate the negative consequences of social situations.

For someone to be diagnosed with a social anxiety disorder, the disturbance must be experienced across a range of situations, rather than a single setting (such as public speaking), and significantly interfere with everyday routines, work, school, and interpersonal relationships.

Social anxiety disorder is usually accompanied by anticipatory worry (worry that occurs in advance) and associated behaviors that include avoidance.

Phobias

A phobia is a persistent, excessive, irrational fear of a specific object, activity, or situation that actually poses little or no danger. A phobia is typically evoked nearly every time someone comes in contact with the thing they fear. Individuals actively avoid this thing, and if they are unable to avoid it, the situation evokes intense fear or anxiety. Some phobias are specific and limited, while others relate to a wider variety of stimuli.

The American Psychiatric Association identifies three primary types of phobias:

- Specific phobia (such as fear of heights, snakes, or spiders)
- Social phobia (such as using public restrooms or eating in front of others)
- Agoraphobia (discomfort in situations where escape feels restricted or help is not readily available)

Most phobias develop in early childhood, and typically the first experience that an individual has with a phobia is a panic attack.

Panic Attacks

A panic attack is a sudden surge of intense fear or discomfort that reaches a peak within a short period (usually within minutes), which is either expected (anticipated and related to a particular stimulus) or unexpected (out of the blue with no obvious cue or trigger at the time of occurrence). Panic attacks are accompanied by physical and cognitive symptoms such as heart palpitations, shortness of breath, dizziness, trembling, and fears of dying, going crazy, or losing control.

Panic attacks are also accompanied by intense worry about the prospect of future attacks and the physical (having a heart attack or a seizure), social (being embarrassed or judged), and mental (going crazy or losing control) functioning consequences. Individuals usually adopt maladaptive or restrictive changes in their behavior to avoid panic attacks and their consequences (such as avoiding physical exertion or reorganizing daily life).

A panic disorder is characterized by recurrent and unexpected, full-symptom panic attacks.

Worry

While not a disorder, worry forms the foundation of several anxiety disorders, particularly generalized anxiety.

Common worry allows us to think ahead, anticipate problems, and plan future events where outcomes are uncertain. However, excessive or pathological worry is often described as a chain of thoughts and images, overloaded with negativity and appearing relatively uncontrollable.

Worry is future tense (such as, "What if something terrible happens?") and differs significantly from rumination, which is excessive thoughts about past events or negative personal attributes (such as, "Why am I such a failure?"). Anticipating the possibility of danger may have served our ancestors, but it is uncertain why we worry excessively when the probability of danger is so low—worry tends to cause distress without any real value. Our brains have not quite evolved from when we huddled around the fire at night for protection.

Clinically, excessive worry is the primary symptom of a generalized anxiety disorder.

The Anxiety Index

This brief self-assessment guide can help you identify potential anxiety-related conditions. Your answers to the questions on the next few pages will serve as a reference for using this workbook and guide the direction and nature of your treatment. The index is a list of symptoms commonly associated with anxiety-related disorders.

Instructions: Carefully read each question and answer them to the best of your ability. Once you have completed the anxiety index, complete the "Self-Assessment" box on page 19.

Generalized Anxiety Index Symptom Descriptions	YES	or	NO
Do you experience fear or anxiety that creates significant distress or impairment in social, occupational, or other daily functioning areas?	☐		☐
Is the fear or anxiety persistent (for six months or more)?	☐		☐
Is the fear or anxiety out of proportion to the threat posed?	☐		☐
Is there a possibility that your symptoms are signaling another potential condition? (If Yes, it is highly recommended to consult with your primary care physician.)	☐		☐
Is there a possibility that your symptoms are caused by some form of substance or medication? (If Yes, it is highly recommended to consult with your primary care physician.)	☐		☐

Specific Anxiety Index Symptom Descriptions

SPECIFIC PHOBIAS   **YES** or **NO**

Is there a distinct increase in fear or anxiety associated   ☐   ☐
with a specific object or situation (such as flying, heights,
or animals)?

Does the identified thing almost always trigger immediate   ☐   ☐
fear or anxiety?

Is there an active avoidance or attempt to endure the object   ☐   ☐
or situation that evokes intense fear or anxiety?

SOCIAL ANXIETY DISORDER   **YES** or **NO**

Is there fear or anxiety about one or more social situations in   ☐   ☐
which there is exposure to possible scrutiny by others?

Is there fear of displaying anxiety symptoms that will be neg-   ☐   ☐
atively evaluated (that will be humiliating or embarrassing,
lead to rejection, or offend others)?

Does the social situation almost always provoke fear   ☐   ☐
or anxiety?

Are social situations avoided or endured with intense fear   ☐   ☐
or anxiety?

PANIC DISORDER

Check off any symptoms that you have experienced:

☐ Palpitations or pounding heart   ☐ Chills or heat sensations
☐ Sweating, shaking, or trembling   ☐ Numbness or tingling sensations
☐ Shortness of breath or sensa-   ☐ Feelings of being detached
   tions of choking   ☐ Worry about losing control or
☐ Chest pain or tightness   "going crazy"
☐ Nausea or abdominal pain   ☐ Fear of dying
☐ Dizziness, lightheadedness, or
   feeling faint

Is there an experience of repeat unexpected panic attacks that occur with an abrupt surge of intense fear or discomfort that reaches a peak within a few minutes, and that is accompanied by four or more of the above symptoms? (Note: The abrupt surge can occur from a calm or anxious state.) ☐ ☐

Has there been an occurrence of a panic attack in the past month that also included the presence of one or more of these symptoms? ☐ ☐

Have you experienced ongoing worry about additional panic attacks or fear about the consequences (such as losing control, having a heart attack, or "going crazy")? ☐ ☐

Have you experienced negative avoidant behavior brought on by an attack? ☐ ☐

Self-Assessment

In the box below, write down what you believe could be the anxiety-related disturbance or experience you have been struggling with.

I believe I have been struggling with:

Note: This index does not constitute or replace a formal clinical assessment and diagnosis. For a thorough and more accurate assessment and proper diagnosis of a mental health concern, it is highly recommended to seek professional medical advice.

It Will Get Better

Many men have been living with anxiety for so long, they are unable to differentiate themselves from it. It's a constant companion that was never invited or welcome. The great news is that you are not your anxiety, and you are not stuck with it. It is well within your reach to live a life in which anxiety no longer has a debilitating hold over you.

Imagine being able to go to sleep at night without replaying everything you did or rehashing conversations you had during the day, over and over in your head. Imagine having the ability to comfortably attend social events, exercise at the gym, or feel at ease at work. You can manage your anxiety for good, instead of turning to the temporary crutches of anger, isolation, or substance abuse to mute the worry and doubt.

Scores of men have successfully overcome anxiety and gone on to live peaceful and fulfilling lives. They have adopted many of the tools in this workbook and blazed a distinct path for other men to follow so they, too, can realize their fullest potential. And now you can undertake this journey for yourself.

When men engage in therapeutic work to address their anxiety, they often realize:

- Anxiety does not define who they are.
- There is nothing inherently wrong or broken about them.
- There is always hope.

Because you're the expert on your life with anxiety, describe what life would be like without it. Imagine you woke up into a life without the burden of anxiety:

- As you open your eyes on this new day, what is different?
- How can you tell things have changed for the better?
- What is different from the way you felt before?
- What will you do throughout this new day that you couldn't do before?

It's important to remember that typical anxiety does serve us in many positive ways and will never disappear completely. However, the debilitating impact it has had on you can be conquered. The life you just imagined is well within your reach!

Debrief & Digest

We've covered a lot in this first chapter, so let's take a moment to digest it all:

- We examined how men process, deal with, and convey their anxiety, particularly through substance use or abuse, anger, irritability, depression, and suicidal ideation.

- We explored the impact of social norms and stigmas preventing men from seeking therapeutic support.
- We looked at the construct of anxiety, including environmental and genetic factors, as well as the role of worry and various forms of anxiety: generalized anxiety disorder, social anxiety disorder, phobias, and panic disorder.

The stage is set for the practical work that lies ahead. As with any new undertaking, the first step is always the most challenging. I applaud your courage. At the end of each chapter, we'll do a quick check-in. Let's kick that off here.

Chapter Check-In

Take a few moments to answer the following questions:

- What are the potential upsides for you in continuing to use this workbook to explore and conquer anxiety?

- What have you started to discover about yourself and your experience of anxiety from reading this chapter?

- What additional information or guidance would you like in order to manage anxiety and experience calm and clarity in your life?

CHAPTER 2

Get Familiar with Your Anxiety

It's hard to fix what you can't find or don't understand. This chapter aims to help you shine a light on the unique causes and symptoms of your anxiety so you can develop a personalized treatment plan.

In this chapter, you'll begin to understand which unique triggers evoke your fear, anxiety, and stress and examine the potential areas of your life that could be adversely impacted by anxiety. Finally, you will be invited to create a clear goal that focuses on reducing anxiety and improving your overall well-being.

Anxiety Triggers

To have a solid shot at managing your emotions and finding a sense of calm, it'll take some forensic work and courage to learn about and disarm these disruptive feelings.

Anxiety can feel like it comes out of nowhere, but it typically occurs when certain stimuli or "triggers" are activated within us. These distressing triggers result in a cognitive, emotional, physical, and/or behavioral response that keeps us stuck in a cycle of anxiety. Because we all have unique memories and experiences, the stimuli that activate anxiety are highly personal and subjective.

While we don't know precisely how triggers are formed, some schools of thought believe our brain and body store "memories" from past traumatic events and refer to them when stimulated. However, the exact functioning behind such triggers is not fully understood.

Learning to identify our unique triggers is the first major step in diffusing anxiety. Understanding which stimuli or triggers influence you begins by understanding some of the potential areas of life that evoke anxiety for many men, including social and interpersonal interactions, education, career, health and well-being, and everyday responsibilities.

Awareness and knowledge are the foundations for identifying our anxiety and implementing a solution. Being able to objectively observe our triggers and gain insight into the origins of these emotions can be tough, especially while we are in the throes of anxiety. Hang in there, and know that you'll learn to develop these skills as you use the tools throughout this book.

Let's take a closer look at some common domains where anxiety likes to hide out.

Social Interactions

At our core, we are social creatures. We desire to connect with others, build intimate relationships, and, ultimately, be liked. Positive interactions can boost confidence and self-esteem, making us feel loved and worthy. Conversely, an inability to smoothly navigate social interactions can lead to feelings of anger, shame, hopelessness, isolation, and depression.

Anxiety can play out in many awkward and uncomfortable ways in the context of social and intimate relationships. Just as experiencing relationship conflicts can induce anxiety, anxiety can also be an underlying cause for why social interactions go awry.

When struggling to build meaningful relationships, we may encounter anxiety-inducing characteristics such as difficulty expressing emotions, trouble attending to the needs and fears of others, feeling defensive, or difficulty experiencing joy. Emotions like shyness, irritability or impatience, and a tendency to be judgmental of others can also impair our ability to connect. Even being unable to read a room or a nonverbal expression can pose monumental barriers to communication.

With so many ways anxiety can make things weird, it's a wonder any of us are able to build meaningful connections! Still, identifying your past challenges with social interactions will help you navigate similar situations in the future.

Education or Career

The first question men typically ask one another is "What do you do?" Perhaps this is because men often derive self-esteem, identity, and personal happiness from their work.

While impressive job titles and advanced degrees may be markers for the external status men crave, it can be especially hard for men with anxiety to reach their full potential. Low workplace productivity, absenteeism, and poor relationships with peers, teachers, or employers are just some of the hurdles that stem from anxiety. At work, those with anxiety may also have trouble concentrating, focus on the fear instead of work, excessively self-focus, and turn down opportunities because of a fear of failure and procrastination.

When it comes to school, anxiety negatively influences academic progress and achievement. Students with high anxiety sometimes score lower on IQ and achievement tests than their peers because of procrastination and worry.

Health and Well-Being

Well-being is a term that encompasses how you feel and function, on both a personal and a social level, and how you evaluate your life. Objectively, there may be things in your life that are challenging, but it's how you feel about those challenges that have the biggest impact on your life.

Anxiety can adversely impact all aspects of well-being and can be especially damaging to our sense of co-vitality. Co-vitality is our overall perception of well-being. The areas of co-vitality most affected by anxiety are hope, optimism, grit, self-efficacy, life satisfaction, happiness, and gratitude—in simple terms, our perspective regarding our quality of life and our life experiences.

Acting as a filter on our experiences, anxiety can make it hard to see the good and exacerbate the bad, challenging every aspect of our well-being.

Everyday Responsibilities

Anxiety can be exhausting, often present from the moment you rise until you finally fall asleep at night. Gnawing thoughts of fear and worry can make the simplest tasks of daily living extra taxing, like getting ready for work or facing common social interactions.

While the occurrence and severity can vary from person to person, often those who struggle with chronic anxiety say that small, everyday trials and tribulations make anxiety hard to endure.

Often, men with anxiety worry about things that could possibly go wrong, or they stew over past interactions or events that didn't go well, leading to self-criticism, procrastination, and fear of failure.

The ability to make simple decisions can be impaired by anxiety. Envisioning irrational or "worst case" scenarios dominates and paralyzes decision-making. As a result, it feels impossible for some individuals to get through the tasks of the day.

Developing Trigger Awareness

Identifying triggers that activate anxiety is an important step toward developing and adopting positive tactics to create calm. This exercise introduces the tactic of self-monitoring.

Think about the last time your anxiety was elevated. Use the table on the next page to list the triggers that may have evoked anxiety and the degree of intensity that you experienced on a scale of 1 to 10 (10 being the highest degree of anxiety). Finally, write down the thoughts, feelings, and physical and behavioral response that you then experienced.

Use this table to record five triggers that you can recall, and/or use it to monitor any triggers you might experience as you progress through this workbook.

TRIGGER TYPE (OBJECT/SITUATION/ PERSON/MEMORY)	DEGREE OF ANXIETY INTENSITY	TRIGGER RESPONSE
Situation: Presentation to my work colleagues.	6/10	**Thought:** Imagining my boss thinks I'm underprepared.
		Physical: Feeling flushed, tight chest.
		Behavior: I withdrew and went quiet.

→

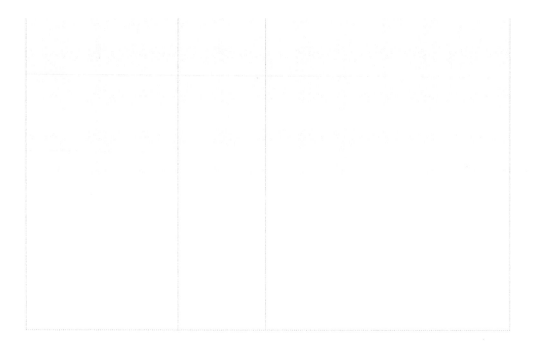

As with any skill, the more self-monitoring you do, the better you'll become. The aim is to eventually self-monitor in real time. You'll learn more about self-monitoring in chapter 3.

What's Going On?

"It is a capital mistake to theorize before you have all the evidence. It biases the judgment."

—Sherlock Holmes

It can take a bit of detective work to figure out the underlying causes of your anxiety. Luckily, there's no one who knows more about your symptoms than you! Building awareness around your anxiety allows you to "reverse engineer," or work backward to get to the source. This method of deductive reasoning is part of a simple yet effective strategy for alleviating most mental health concerns.

It's important to examine the role of cause and effect. By defining your triggers and noticing when and where they arise, you can learn if your anxiety is occurring because of an internal stimulus or as a reflection of what's happening to you in a given moment (something in your environment). This is an essential distinction in managing anxiety, because it can be challenging to determine whether the stimuli or triggers you experience are the underlying causes of anxiety or merely the associated consequences of the stimuli—the latter often perpetuating the problem.

Think about a microphone placed too close to an amplifier. We experience the ear-splitting noise from the speakers, and we focus immediately on addressing the pain it causes to our hearing. However, break the negative feedback cycle (move the microphone to a safe distance) and the noise stops.

In the next exercise, we'll use four action steps to observe your experience with anxiety: explore, evaluate, prepare, and act. Using these action steps, we'll explore three domains commonly experienced with anxiety: physical, cognitive, and behavioral symptoms.

Observing the Experience of Anxiety

Over the next few days, set aside a few minutes each day to reflect on your most recent anxiety experience. You can also refer back to this exercise over the next few days and record your thoughts as anxious, worrisome, or fearful moments occur. Write as much detail about your experience as possible.

• Describe the various ways that anxiety was experienced or expressed, such as physical symptoms, feelings, thoughts, and actions that occurred.

....

....

....

• Reflect on the consequences of this experience. What problems did it cause? What problems does anxiety generally cause in your life that were reflected in this instance?

....

....

- Describe the various domains of your life that are potentially impacted. Consider relationships with friends and family, work and school pursuits, and financial, spiritual, recreational, health, and fitness goals.

  ....

  ....

- Describe what about the experience you most disliked.

  ....

  ....

- What is the worst thing about being anxious, worried, or fearful?

  ....

- What were the advantages of experiencing anxiety?

  ....

  ....

- What were the disadvantages of experiencing anxiety?

  ....

  ....

Some readers might find themselves triggered by reading the anecdotes presented in each of the following sections. If you experience a heightened sense of anxiety while reading these examples, please feel free to skip and return to these sections later or use the CALM tool (see page 34).

Physical Symptoms

Khanh just finished a long day at work, and he was looking forward to getting home. There wasn't too much traffic. He stopped at a red light. Without any warning, Khanh suddenly started to feel overwhelmed. His cheeks started to flush, and he felt a hot sensation envelop his body. His hands on the steering wheel seemed cold. His heart began to race, and it felt like it was about to explode out of his chest. The world around him was spinning and he feared he would lose control of the car, even though he knew he was stationary. He struggled to inhale, and gasped for air. He managed to switch on his hazard lights and turn off the engine. He placed his head on the steering wheel and remained there for about 10 minutes. Eventually, his nausea and fear subsided and he gained perspective about his surroundings. His muscles ached like he had just finished an intense workout. He started his car and managed to make his way home safely.

This scenario represents the experience of an unexpected panic attack. Of all the symptoms to be explored and examined, physical symptoms can be the easiest for men to recognize. They can be instant, overwhelming, and undeniable.

A wide range of physical responses can occur during a panic attack, including:

- Hyperventilation: rapid breathing, shortness of breath, sweating, chills, cold/clammy hands, paling, flushing
- A cardiovascular system response: pounding heart or increased heart rate, chest pain, increased blood pressure
- A somatic (body) response: difficulty speaking, dizziness, nausea, abdominal distress

This fight-or-flight response can be extremely useful if you're being chased by a tiger or have to swerve around an oncoming car, but without any apparent danger in sight, it can feel upsetting, confusing, and without sense. The good news is there are effective ways to work through this, which we'll explore later in this book.

- Reflect on your last experience of anxiety. Close your eyes. Scan your body from head to toe, connecting with each part. What are you feeling now?

- Reflect on the physical symptoms you associate with your most recent experience of anxiety. What do you recognize? Write down the symptoms you identify. What was happening before, during, or immediately after you recognized these symptoms?

Cognitive Symptoms

Alex plucked up the courage to go on a blind date. He sat at a table in an elegant restaurant. While he was waiting for his date to arrive, his thoughts started to wander. He worried about whether the person he was about to meet would find him attractive, and he imagined them turning and walking away the moment they saw him. A persistent thought, "Don't blow this one. You never have any success with dating," bounced around his head. "Maybe they won't come. Maybe I'm just not cut out for dating." The negative thoughts picked up speed, and he started to spiral. The room began to shrink. He felt as though others seated around him were judging him. He felt inadequate and fearful of what might happen when his date arrived. It was proving to be more challenging to remain in control. "Keep it together," he muttered. Because he was so deep in thought, he failed to recognize that his date was standing in front of him.

As humans, we possess the brilliant gift of cognition. Our mind helps us navigate through every life experience using processes that assist with attention, perception, pattern recognition, memory, reasoning, problem-solving, decision-making, knowledge representation, imagination, and language.

However, anxiety has a pesky way of altering or limiting our cognitive processes. This limitation, called "cognitive distortion," has adverse consequences on our ability to interact with the world around us, and influences how we view ourselves.

Different types of anxiety, such as social anxiety disorder or panic attack disorder, present different cognitive symptoms. The scenario you just read highlights some cognitive symptoms typical of social anxiety. These include negative interpretations or predictions (jumping to conclusions) coupled with negative self-demands (should/must statements) about how one should act, as well as visual disorientation and dissociation (a state of separation from the present situation).

- Take a moment to reflect on the thoughts or images that occurred during your last experience of anxiety. What do you recall?

....

....

- Write down what was happening before, during, or immediately after you recognized these symptoms.

....

....

Behavioral Symptoms

Lewis was invited to a social gathering where he was unfamiliar with a number of the people present. This was not the first time he had felt out of place, and he frequently struggled to start conversations with people he didn't know. He often didn't know what to say. As the evening progressed, Lewis found the stress of interacting with others increasing, and the pressure kept growing. To numb his nerves, Lewis started to drink heavily. As he became more intoxicated, Lewis became verbally and physically aggressive toward several fellow guests. There was an altercation, and Lewis was asked to leave.

Anxiety can significantly influence our behavior, especially when it involves reacting with a fight response or a flight response. Also, in an attempt to numb or disconnect from anxiety, many men will adopt unhealthy behaviors such as substance use or other risky or harmful practices.

In chapter 1, we explored the various anxiety disorders (see page 14). The following are common behavioral responses for each of the anxiety disorders, as described by the DSM-5:

Generalized anxiety disorder (GAD): Key behaviors include persistent worry, a behavior that aims to pursue a desired outcome or avoid stress.

Social anxiety disorder (SAD): A typical response is to avoid social interactions and situations that involve the possibility of being scrutinized. Those who struggle with SAD will adopt a wide range of avoidant or pursuant behaviors, such as being inordinately assertive or excessively submissive. Many display shyness or withdrawal and may even avoid or delay establishing intimate relationships, marrying, and having a family.

Panic disorder: A common response is to use avoidance in an attempt to reduce the likelihood of a panic attack recurring.

Phobia: An obvious response is to actively minimize contact with phobic objects or situations.

- Take a moment to reflect on the behaviors that you associate with your last experience of anxiety. What do you identify?

  ....

  ....

- What was happening before, during, or immediately after you recognized these responses?

  ....

  ....

In the Moment

For men who have struggled with anxiety and are looking for ways to navigate it, it's essential to have a "break glass in case of an emergency" plan. This simple tool is helpful when you need to regulate and focus yourself when you are experiencing anxiety symptoms. It's called CALM, which stands for center, affirm, locate, and move. Here's how it works:

Center and reclaim control of your body, mind, and behavior. Centering can include mindfulness practices or deep relaxation techniques such as structured breathing and muscle relaxation. Choose one of the structured breathing practices from chapter 8 to assist with centering and have it ready.

Affirm that you can manage anxiety successfully and that you're worthy of the things you envision for yourself. Affirmations are a valuable tool for restructuring negative thoughts and beliefs. Prepare an affirmation for yourself and have it ready to repeat aloud when anxious. Write your affirmation on the line provided. Examples might include:

I am not my anxiety.

This, too, shall pass.

My fears are merely paper tigers; they are not real.

....

Locate yourself in the present and not the future. Anxiety is future-focused, so reminding ourselves to be "in the moment" or "in the here and now" is hugely beneficial. Engage your senses to help. What can you touch, see, or hear that will bring you into the present?

....

....

Move intentionally. This allows us to discharge stress hormones from our body, which flood us during elevated anxiety. Gentle, purposeful activity such as walking or slow stretching helps significantly with creating calm.

Set Your Goals

"Success is the progressive realization of a worthy goal
or ideal."

—Earl Nightingale

Clear, concrete goals can help us reach our preferred destination. Goals provide the road map on which to focus our attention, time, and energy. They help us navigate forward when things get difficult, because change never occurs in a straight line.

Let's establish a road map for your goals. It can include both short-term and long-term goals. This is an important differentiation, because most men who struggle with anxiety will often have immediate symptoms they need to address, as well as challenges that may not be apparent at the time.

You've already spent some time imagining what life would be like without anxiety. You've also spent a bit of time exploring the principal symptoms of your anxiety. Here, you'll be using this knowledge to construct a series of intentions.

Step 1: Set an intention

Ask yourself, "When I am successful in managing my anxiety and I experience calm on a daily basis, what are three things that will have changed for the better?"

Write down three things to focus on incrementally that will have a positive impact. Start small and work toward bigger intentions as you go.

Here's an example: *When I am successful in managing my anxiety, I will be able to maintain a sense of calm when interacting with my work colleagues (first area of focus). I will worry less about what others think about me in social environments (second area of focus), and I will be more confident in initiating new social and professional connections (third area of focus).*

Step 2: Get specific

Write down the physical, cognitive, and behavioral symptoms that will decrease when you are successful in managing your anxiety. For example:

- **Physical:** reduced sweating, decreased heart rate, no vomiting
- **Cognitive:** reduced negative self-talk, not jumping to conclusions
- **Behavioral:** reduced avoidance of others and decreased negative rumination

Physical:

Cognitive:

Behavioral:

Physical:

Cognitive:

Behavioral:

Physical:

Cognitive:

Behavioral:

Step 3: Expand your intention

Let's work on expanding your intentions using the SMART analogy. SMART is a widely referenced approach to goal-setting. It refers to a goal that is specific, measurable, achievable, relevant, and timely. Write your SMART goal in the space provided.

Example: *It is my intention to successfully achieve a sense of calm when interacting with my work colleagues* (specific). *I will measure the achievement of this goal by documenting the number of times I experience calmness and serenity when engaging* (measurable). *I will decrease my negative self-talk and avoidant behavior, which is the initial strategy of my long-term goal of overcoming anxiety* (achievable). *This goal is important because my anxiety has affected my work performance* (relevant). *I will measure my progress over the next four weeks* (timely).

Debrief & Digest

There's a lot of information in this chapter, so it's natural to feel a little mentally overloaded. Keep up the great work—it does get easier.

- We've identified the various anxiety-related triggers men experience, so you are now more prepared to spot and monitor your own triggers when they occur. By deepening your awareness, you were able to explore the physical, cognitive, and behavioral symptoms that accompany your anxiety.
- We've considered the various areas in life that can be adversely impacted by anxiety, including social and interpersonal relationships, education and career pursuits, overall health and well-being, and general daily responsibilities.
- Most important, you've used all that knowledge and awareness to establish a self-treatment plan to act as your guide as you adopt the tips, tools, and tactics in this workbook.

Chapter Check-In

To digest all you've learned, take a few moments to answer the following questions:

- What are the main triggers you've identified that evoke anxiety for you?

  ....

  ....

  ....

- What symptoms are most prevalent when you experience anxiety? What were you already familiar with, and what new symptoms did you become aware of?

  ....

  ....

  ....

- What skills, knowledge, or experiences do you already possess that could be harnessed to successfully manage anxiety?

  ....

  ....

  ....

- What barriers or obstacles could potentially impede or restrict your ability to achieve the goal you created?

  ....

  ....

  ....

CHAPTER 3

Managing Your Anxiety

Now that you've examined your personal experience of anxiety and its potential root causes, let's look at some models for creating calm in your life.

First, we'll look at the "gold standard" of psychotherapy, cognitive behavioral therapy (CBT), and discuss why it is commonly used in the treatment of anxiety-related disorders, including panic disorder and social anxiety disorder. We'll also look at specific CBT techniques such as mindfulness and meditation practices, acceptance and commitment therapy (ACT), and clinical hypnotherapy.

Cognitive Behavioral Therapy

Building awareness around the triggers and symptoms of your anxiety is imperative. It might feel challenging, but this is the first step and the foundation of all future work. From here, we will dig in and employ the most direct and successful techniques for resolving it: cognitive behavioral therapy (CBT), a short-term, goal-oriented form of psychotherapy that involves a practical approach to problem-solving.

The main components that make up CBT include psychoeducation about the nature of fear and anxiety, self-monitoring of symptoms, somatic (body) exercises, cognitive restructuring (challenging and changing negative thinking), exposure to feared stimuli, and relapse prevention. You've already done some of this work with what you've learned and explored so far, and we'll continue in the coming chapters.

CBT tackles anxiety from two directions. From a cognitive perspective, it explores and challenges cognitive distortions that perpetuate the cycle of anxiety. From a behavioral perspective, CBT supports actions that disrupt the cycle of anxiety. Collectively, this dual focus helps improve emotional and physical regulation.

The best part: It's very successful! Research indicates that one year after treatment, up to 62 percent of participants continued to meet criteria for positive outcome results. Additionally, up to 77 percent of participants who used CBT for general anxiety disorders maintained relief from their prior symptoms post-treatment.

Why CBT?

Regardless of the problem, the basic principle behind any type of therapy is always the same: How we feel, what we think, and how we behave are interconnected. And all of these factors have a significant influence on our well-being.

As research shows, CBT is highly effective and efficient. CBT is built on the theory that our general beliefs about the world, the self, and the future evoke specific and automatic thoughts in particular situations. More specifically, this approach maintains that it's not events themselves that create problems, but the meaning we assign to these events. CBT fosters active participation in exploring, challenging, and altering maladaptive thoughts and beliefs that create the filter through which we perceive our experiences.

One of the most appealing aspects of CBT is that while other forms of therapy may focus on childhood influences or more existential concerns, CBT is goal-oriented, problem-focused, and time-structured, meaning it doesn't drag out indefinitely. The tools you gain using CBT to resolve anxiety are also useful for solving future problems.

How Does It Work?

CBT starts with learning how to identify maladaptive thoughts, beliefs, and behaviors that trigger and sustain the symptoms of anxiety.

For example, imagine if you failed a task at work, and an involuntary thought or idea popped into your head that says, *I can't do anything right*. This thought might lead to a particular reaction. You might feel sad (emotion) and retreat or withdraw (behavior). When a pattern like this is repeated day after day, it cultivates an anxiety response that can be difficult to disrupt.

To counteract this type of automatic anxiety response, CBT focuses on a deeper level of cognition, which includes your basic beliefs about yourself, your world, and other people. Working to shift your thinking about these underlying dysfunctional beliefs can change your perception of situations that trigger anxiety. And this change in perception produces more enduring change. Throughout the CBT process, individuals learn to become acutely aware of the triggers and symptoms that evoke anxiety and how to adopt positive "triggers" that result in more desirable cognitive and behavioral outcomes. Different anxiety disorders may respond better to different CBT approaches, which have all been developed over the past few decades.

For example, CBT models that address generalized and social anxiety disorders focus on worry metacognitions (the thinking of thinking), difficulty managing emotions, and acceptance-based strategies. Other anxiety-related disorders work to target uncertainty, excessive worry, negative views toward perceived problems or challenges, and cognitive avoidance, which is avoiding unwanted or intrusive thoughts. A trusted therapist can help determine which techniques will be most beneficial.

Exploring Your Options

Take a moment to think about what you've just learned about cognitive behavioral therapy. Answer the following questions, then reflect on your answers.

How important is it to achieve your goal of successfully managing anxiety and experiencing calm in your life?

- ☐ Not at all important
- ☐ Slightly important
- ☐ Important
- ☐ Somewhat important
- ☐ Very important

How willing are you to use CBT to achieve the goal you established for yourself?

- ☐ Not at all willing or interested
- ☐ Slightly willing
- ☐ Willing
- ☐ Somewhat willing
- ☐ Very willing

How confident are you about adopting CBT to manage anxiety and experience calm?

- ☐ Not at all confident
- ☐ Slightly confident
- ☐ Confident
- ☐ Somewhat confident
- ☐ Very confident

Other Types of Treatment

Many therapists don't tie themselves to any one approach, because no one therapeutic model fits all (such as just using CBT on its own). Instead, they blend elements from different approaches and tailor their treatment according to each individual's needs. This is described as integrative or holistic therapy.

A psychotherapist will consider the nature of the problem, the person's readiness and ability to engage in therapy, and the individual's personality in order to establish an effective treatment plan.

Therapy may also include the integration of psychotherapy and psychiatric medications, as psychiatric medications are usually more effective when combined with psychotherapy. In some cases, medication can reduce symptoms so other treatment plans can be more effective. In these instances, a psychotherapist will collaborate with other mental health specialists, such as a psychiatrist.

Other psychotherapy-related options include acceptance and commitment therapy (ACT), exposure therapy, biofeedback, and clinical hypnotherapy. Additional tools such as mindfulness and meditation practices are also widely accepted and frequently incorporated into treatment choices for anxiety. Let's take a closer look at these.

Mindfulness and Meditation

Mindfulness is the practice of paying attention to what is happening in the present moment. It's an important tool in developing awareness about the triggers and symptoms commonly associated with anxiety. Mindfulness can reduce stress, promote an increased sense of well-being, and decrease depression and anxiety. It reduces rumination and overthinking and supports positive emotional reactivity and cognitive flexibility (open-mindedness)—all significantly associated with anxiety.

Mindfulness encompasses two main things: awareness and acceptance. Awareness is the ability to focus your attention on your inner processes and experiences in the present moment. Acceptance is the ability to observe and accept your thoughts as they come, rather than judging or avoiding them—this is particularly helpful during meditation.

Meditation is used to increase physical relaxation, improve psychological balance, and enhance overall health and well-being. This is achieved through intentionally resting the mind and breathing.

Acceptance and Commitment Therapy

Acceptance and commitment therapy (ACT; pronounced like "act") is a therapeutic model that combines acceptance and mindfulness strategies with commitment and behavior-change strategies to increase cognitive flexibility. ACT stands for accepting thoughts and feelings, choosing directions, and taking action.

It encourages individuals to embrace their thoughts, feelings, and experiences, rather than fight against them. ACT attempts to transform our relationship with our difficult thoughts and feelings to no longer perceive them as "symptoms" but as harmless passing experiences. It also normalizes and views the experience of anxiety with compassion and understanding.

Exposure Therapy

Exposure therapy is intentional exposure to the things that evoke fear, as a way to desensitize the individual to the object, experience, or situation that they attempt to avoid. Avoidance offers the individual immediate or temporary relief; however, ironically, it prolongs and exacerbates anxiety in the long term.

In exposure therapy, a safe environment is created to expose individuals to the things they fear and avoid. This exposure in a safe environment helps reduce fear and decreases avoidance. When forced to repeatedly confront a fear, the mind essentially adapts to the stimulus that causes that fear and stops finding it stressful.

Scientifically, exposure therapy is shown to be a helpful treatment component for phobias, panic disorder, social anxiety disorder, obsessive-compulsive disorder (OCD), post-traumatic stress disorder (PTSD), and generalized anxiety disorder.

Biofeedback

Biofeedback is a self-regulation technique through which patients learn to voluntarily control what they once believed to be involuntary body processes. It typically involves an EEG, a procedure that provides neurological or biological feedback through the use of sensors placed on the patient's skin.

These sensors can monitor an individual's physiological state and feed information about it back to that person. This feedback helps the participant consciously control aspects of their physiology using relaxation and mindfulness techniques. By doing this, the participant can slow down the sympathetic nervous system and heart rate, a significant factor in managing anxiety. Biofeedback helps facilitate subtle changes in the body, such as relaxing specific muscles to reduce pain, improve a health condition, or optimize physical performance.

Biofeedback is a form of mental and physical training. Rather than passively receiving treatment, the patient is an active learner and understands more about how the body functions and how it can be managed to create optimal well-being.

Clinical Hypnotherapy

Clinical hypnotherapy is a tool that can treat a wide range of issues such as fear, phobias, anxiety, stress, panic attacks, and insomnia. The American Society of Clinical Hypnosis defines hypnosis as "a state of consciousness involving focused attention and reduced peripheral awareness characterized by an enhanced capacity for response to suggestion."

For the treatment of anxiety, hypnotherapy is highly effective in creating a heightened state of awareness and increasing the receptibility of the mind for exploration and suggestion. This means that individuals can move through the natural resistance that is sometimes experienced in therapy, increasing the effectiveness and timeliness of treatment. Research suggests that an integrated approach combining clinical hypnosis and CBT increases the efficacy of treatment.

Committing to the Journey

Developing the discipline required to be successful in achieving goals can be aided by answering several crucial questions along the way.

- What's the underpinning motivation for you to navigate and manage anxiety?

  _____

  _____

  _____

  _____

- What guidance would you offer to a close friend if they embarked on a similar journey?

  _____

  _____

  _____

  _____

- What will your life look like 10 weeks, 10 months, or 10 years from now, once you have successfully achieved your goal?

  _____

  _____

  _____

  _____

Debrief & Digest

In this chapter:

- We dove into the prominent psychotherapeutic model for resolving anxiety disorders: cognitive behavioral therapy.
- We explored other various psychotherapy models that are considered effective in supporting awareness of the causes and influences of anxiety, as well as tactics that help develop calm and address fear and worry.

As you proceed through the rest of this workbook, you'll learn in more detail some pivotal tools and techniques that each of these models offers to assist you in managing anxiety.

Ready for the exciting part? We've hit a major turning point, where we move beyond understanding and awareness and focus on taking action. Before you embark on the next chapter, reflect on what you've learned with the following exercise.

Chapter Check-In

Well done on all the heavy lifting! Working through how to manage anxiety is not an easy task. Let's sign off by exploring the meaning of anxiety and how it may have shaped your world so far.

- What meaning have you assigned to the experience of anxiety?

  _____

  _____

  _____

  _____

- What would it mean to you if you were to successfully manage anxiety and experience calm and confidence?

  _____

  _____

....

....

- What thoughts about the world, yourself, and anxiety do you think you might be referencing during stressful or challenging situations that trigger anxiety?

....

....

....

....

- What would happen if you successfully challenged and altered negative thoughts of the things you worry about?

....

....

....

....

CHAPTER 4

Recognize & Challenge Negative Thinking

We've explored the idea that being able to recognize and challenge the thoughts that occur in anxiety-provoking situations is an important skill to successfully reduce anxiety. In this chapter, you'll be introduced to the negative thinking cycle and some thought patterns that adversely influence how we interpret and respond to ambiguous situations.

You'll have the opportunity to confront thoughts that perpetuate anxiety using practical exercises and tactics, including observing and assessing thoughts for what they really are: simply thoughts.

The Negative Thinking Cycle

One of the predominant experiences of living with anxiety is the constant presence of intrusive or unwanted thoughts. Often, these negative thoughts seem to be stuck in a loop, constantly repeating themselves.

Some thoughts start reasonably innocently, such as worrying whether you'll be able to make a deadline at work or if you closed the garage door when you left the house. But they can amplify and propagate to a point that feels all-consuming. Some thoughts present themselves more like images or video clips, such as imagining friends banishing you from a social gathering or being isolated from others. Oftentimes, negative thoughts generate other unrelated negative thoughts, and they gain their own momentum and direction.

How we think is exceptionally creative, but not always efficient. It's like we have a supercomputer sitting on top of our shoulders containing ineffective code that's causing a software application to freeze and stop working as it's supposed to. Despite hitting Ctrl+Alt+Del, nothing shuts down.

When we engage in any situation, we instantly experience a flood of automatic thoughts. Automatic thoughts are instantaneous, habitual, and unconscious and occur in response to a particular situation or trigger, like "Why does this always happen to me?" or "I know my partner is going to get mad and leave." Some automatic thoughts are apparent. Others are obscured due to other activities going on; that is, our emotions and behavior.

When faulty or negative thinking occurs, there is often an accompanying emotional disturbance, like an instant shift in emotion, such as a state of calm one moment and dread the next. The patterns of faulty or negative thinking that illustrate these emotional disturbances are referred to as *cognitive errors*. These cognitive errors perpetuate and intensify anxiety.

This negative thinking cycle is a form of ineffective mental processing. A situation or stimulus evokes a series of harmful, automatic thoughts, and our reaction to these thoughts leads to adverse emotions and ineffective behaviors. The diagram on page 53, widely used and adapted from Westbrook, Kennerley, and Kirk (2011), illustrates how the negative thinking cycle works.

It is not the situation that determines how we feel or what we do. Rather, it's how we interpret that situation that creates reactions of fear, uncertainty, and doubt. How we interpret experiences is significantly influenced by other cognitive elements. These include primary beliefs, or schemas, which are types of "absolute truths" that we maintain about ourselves, others, and the world around us.

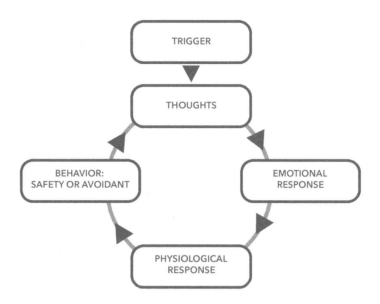

Other cognitive elements include intermediate beliefs, such as values, principles, rules, and assumptions. These beliefs also influence the lens through which we view and interpret an experience. If any of these cognitive elements result in a cognitive error, how we respond to situations will be adversely affected. The end result is a constant state of hypervigilance and anxiety.

All-or-Nothing Thinking

Sebastian has struggled with anxiety since his divorce. His anxiety has increased, and although he's been able to cope for the most part, he is aware of growing thoughts that concern him. Sebastian finds himself thinking in all-or-nothing ways, which leads to moments of poor judgment. He realizes that he's made a number of rash decisions because things feel more urgent and important. Recently, Sebastian found himself in an argument with his new girlfriend. He felt confident about their relationship and knew that she was deeply in love with him, so he asked her to move into his apartment. Unfortunately, she declined. Sebastian started to call himself a "loser" boyfriend and thought he would never be good enough for anyone. His expectations were "ruined," and he felt irritated and deeply disappointed.

A *cognitive distortion* is an automatic, exaggerated, or irrational thought pattern that triggers the onset or perpetuation of anxiety. It's like having a filter over your perception of experiences that causes you to misinterpret what's happening. These distortions may be expressed in a multitude of ways, such as dichotomous, absolute, or catastrophizing thinking.

Dichotomous thinking, also known as all-or-nothing thinking, is an individual's propensity to think in terms of binary opposition, or see things as only good or bad, black or white, right or wrong. This type of binary thinking can help with situations that require quick comprehension or decision-making, such as deciding which way to turn at an intersection or responding to an emergency. However, dichotomous thinking can lead to anxiety when you're faced with more ambiguous or undefined situations.

As we saw with Sebastian, you might say to yourself, "I must get everything right," "If I don't get this job, I'm a failure," or "If my marriage fails, my life is over."

Absolute thinking is another type of cognitive distortion that falls into the dichotomous thought structure. In absolute thinking, words or phrases pop up such as "must," "should," "always," "have to," or "could have" that express a belief that they are responsible for taking one specific or absolute action, and that action holds a certain magnitude or probability.

And catastrophizing is the irrational worrying about potential worst-case scenarios.

The problem with all these types of thinking is that these self-imposed demands or expectations create undue or unrealistic pressure to perform or meet irrational standards. When these expectations aren't met, it can lower self-esteem and self-confidence, perpetuating the cycle of anxiety. However, there are many tools and tactics to help curb these ways of dysfunctional thinking.

Monitoring Your Thoughts

How we harness our thoughts is an essential factor in well-being. Take a moment to reflect on the words that you incorporate into your thinking and verbal communication.

Do you recognize thoughts that use polarized labels or descriptions for certain things, situations, or people—including yourself? For example: "They are evil people," "I'm a deadbeat dad," "I'm either a success or a failure," or "They either love me or they don't." What could be an alternative way to consider the possibilities that lie between these binary labels?

....

....

Do you incorporate absolute thoughts such as "I must," "I need to," "I have to," or "I should"? Do you recognize these as expectations or demands that you place on yourself? What could be a healthier, more realistic way to think about an expectation or desire?

....

....

Write down any absolute thoughts you might say to yourself, as well as an alternative "non-absolute" thought that would work better for you. For example:

Absolute: *I must always be immaculately dressed when I go out.*

Alternative: *It's okay to change up my style from time to time.*

....

....

....

....

Overgeneralizing

When he was six years old, Bryce was bitten by his neighbor's dog. This adverse experience had a significant impact on his experience with other dogs. Even now, as an adult, he avoids dogs and has no interest in owning one. He thinks that dogs simply can't be trusted, and that their owners are often lax when it comes to handling them. Bryce has two young children, and he is extremely vigilant about restricting their interactions with dogs. He says to himself, "It's just a matter of time until one of the kids has a run-in with a dog," and "There are so many terrible reports about careless dog-handling and children being terrorized and attacked." Bryce finds it difficult to believe the positive experiences of those who own dogs, citing that "It's just a matter of time" and that their experiences are simply anomalies or pure luck. Bryce finds himself feeling highly agitated around dogs, and this only validates his thoughts.

Overgeneralizing is another form of cognitive distortion. It is the mental process of making hurried or misguided conclusions without sufficient information or evidence or, like in Bryce's case, as a result of a past experience. Even if something bad happens only once, you now expect that negative situation to happen over and over again.

Overgeneralizing thoughts often refer to situations or experiences in a generic or nonspecific manner. For example, "I don't have what it takes to make friends, and I never will," or "Nobody ever gets a job by doing that," or "People from that profession are unscrupulous and don't have your best interest in mind." You might have gotten sick after eating out at a restaurant the other night, so you conclude that it's much safer to eat at home.

This type of negative thinking is prevalent in panic disorders. Research shows that generalizations can trigger anticipatory anxiety about an unpleasant event recurring. It only makes sense that if you are anxious about something, regardless of whether your fear is based on factual information, you will attempt to avoid that thing or feel anxious about the possibility of encountering it. Overgeneralizing can restrict your ability to learn from past mistakes and tolerate ambiguity and your ability to navigate risk.

An effective approach in conquering overgeneralizations and other forms of dysfunctional thinking is to examine the evidence. Let's try this out.

Examining the Evidence

A practical approach to challenging overgeneralization thinking is to examine the evidence. This requires reflecting on the situation, person, or experience in a more accurate manner. Ask yourself the following questions, and write your answers on the lines provided.

- In what way am I overgeneralizing this situation, experience, or person?

  ....

- What evidence do I have that supports this viewpoint?

  ....

- Is this viewpoint that I hold a verified fact, or is it subjective?

  ....

- What could be an alternative, rational perspective that I could adopt?

  ....

- What impact does dysfunctional thinking have on me, and how does it maintain my anxiety?

  ....

  ....

  ....

Jumping to Conclusions

Jerome was preparing for a job interview with a company that he was excited about joining. He imagined the interview and started to ask himself: "What happens if I stumble over my words, or I fail to answer a question clearly? I know that I'm not cut out for the job, and honestly, it's unlikely that they'll offer it to me." Jerome's thoughts started to spiral, and he began to worry about the worst-case scenario of embarrassing himself and not landing this dream job. If he didn't get this job, he believed, his partner would think he was lazy and incompetent. He imagined life without his partner and envisioned a career doing something monotonous and unfulfilling. Jerome's anxiety elevated, and the emotional and physical symptoms kicked in. Rather than preparing for the interview, he procrastinated by distracting himself with menial tasks around the house.

Jumping to conclusions is one of the most common forms of negative thinking associated with anxiety and worry. This occurs when we arbitrarily make a judgment or decision without accurate or justifiable facts of a situation. The dynamic of jumping to conclusions fails to distinguish between what is observable (fact) and what is assumed (fiction).

While everyone jumps to conclusions sometimes, individuals who experience anxiety often find themselves making interpretations or negative presumptions about a situation. Perhaps you find yourself making unwarranted predictions of potential danger, even though there is no real supporting evidence. This might look like, "If I say no, then that person is going to hate me," or "I'll go to the party, but I know I won't enjoy myself." When this occurs, you might make poor or impulsive choices that could have negative long-term ramifications.

This type of thinking is often applied in novel situations, such as contracting an illness, losing a job, or moving to a new city, where you have limited information available to make decisions. Jumping to conclusions is also used to validate preexisting beliefs. For example, you may think, "My friend will say no if I ask for help, because I believe that asking for help is placing a burden on others." The irony is that if this situation were to occur—a friend saying no to the request even though it had nothing to do with being a burden—it is then used to interpret and confirm your belief to be true. This is called *confirmation bias*.

Other forms of jumping to conclusions include worst-case scenario forecasting, otherwise known as "fortune-telling," where you might envision adverse outcomes or catastrophize a situation.

Mind-reading is another tactic of jumping to conclusions, where you make inferences or assumptions that people are thinking negatively about you, even though there is no evidence. Examples of mind-reading could be "I'm sure they think I'm a jerk for telling that joke," or "I'm sure everyone's thinking I'm a loser sitting here alone in a restaurant."

Recognize When You're Time-Traveling

When we jump to conclusions, it's like we're time-traveling into the future—and just like Marty McFly in *Back to the Future*, we know that time-traveling can be fraught with dangerous consequences. Take a moment to examine whether you adopt this way of thinking, and how that affects you. Answer the following questions in the space provided.

- When faced with a novel or ambiguous situation, what conclusions or inferences do you come up with?

- What do you find yourself thinking or imagining when you worry about what other people might be saying or thinking about you?

- What is the worst-case scenario if the thing you are worrying about were to occur?

- What evidence do you have that supports this thought as true?

  ....

  ....

- On a scale of 1 to 10, what is the likelihood of that experience actually happening?

  1   2   3   4   5   6   7   8   9   10

Confront Your Thoughts

The exact number of thoughts we have on a daily basis is unknown; however, research shows that we spend more time thinking about the future than the past. In fact, one study showed that its participants had 59 future-oriented thoughts per day, which is one future-oriented thought every 16 minutes of the time they were awake.

To gain awareness of and challenge negative, future-oriented thoughts that evoke and prolong symptoms of anxiety, we can look to cognitive behavioral therapy (CBT) for assistance (see page 42). CBT can be used to engage the brain to examine and modify negative thoughts that prevent calm and clarity.

The tools and tactics that CBT uses allow individuals to step back from their thoughts and see them objectively. This process is called *cognitive restructuring*. Cognitive restructuring, or cognitive reframing, is a therapeutic process that helps you discover, challenge, and modify or replace negative, irrational thoughts.

CBT can enable you to break the cycle of negative cognitive, emotional, and behavioral triggers by adopting rational, purposeful thoughts. When these useful thoughts prevail, the result is a positive shift in how you might view and respond to situations that previously evoked anxiety.

Just because a worrisome thought crosses your mind does not make it true or worthy of further examination. Thoughts are just thoughts—they are not facts, messages, predictions, or demands. Try reminding yourself that "thoughts are just thoughts." This incredibly powerful construct prompts us to examine the role that our thoughts might have, including the fact that they are not always valuable or effective.

Fact or Distortion?

Take a moment to reflect on your thoughts about an experience that's either already happened or that you're imagining (future-based). List five to eight thoughts and check whether each thought is factual or if you have adopted a cognitive distortion.

COGNITION/THOUGHT	FACTUAL	DISTORTION
Example: *My colleagues think I'm incompetent.*		✓

Positivity Post-It

Affirmations are brief, positive, intentional statements that can help you challenge and overcome negative thoughts and behaviors. But do they work, or are they too good to be true?

Affirmations offer more than just "feel-good" inspiration—they can be a useful tool for restructuring your thoughts and creating real change. In terms of navigating anxiety, they can help you maintain focus on the various tools, tactics, and constructs for achieving change, as well as your goals.

Affirmations are also helpful for navigating stress, problem-solving, and inspiring creativity. You don't need to be completely convinced that they are working. Just like going to the gym and adopting a new workout program, your body will realize the benefits often before you observe its value. The mind is no different.

Because you are restructuring cognitive processes, there's a lot of activity occurring in the brain. You are actually rewiring the structure of the brain, and, using the same analogy of going to the gym, you are developing muscle memory. In response to any new exercise, there's going to be a bit of natural resistance. Give it some time; it will become easier.

Try this: Write down a brief, positive affirmation on a sticky note or set a recurring reminder in your phone. Use this affirmation to reinforce a desired thought or remind yourself of something you learned in this book. Here are some examples to get you started:

I am not my anxiety.

My thoughts are just thoughts; they are not facts.

I choose to feel calm.

I choose positive and nurturing thoughts.

I am not in danger; I am just uncomfortable. This, too, will pass.

My Thoughts Are Not Me

Thoughts are potent. Whether or not we are consciously aware of them, negative thoughts dramatically influence our brain structure, physiology, emotions, and behavior. The irony is that our thoughts about a situation that evokes anxiety often lead to behavior that confirms our expectations or beliefs. For example, if an individual worries about being rejected by a friend, they may adopt an avoidant behavior like distancing themselves, which leads to the experience of rejection. This phenomenon is referred to as a *self-fulfilling prophecy*, a term used to describe a prediction, expectation, or belief that causes itself to become real.

Thoughts are the output of our cognitive processes. Using the analogy of programming a computer, when we enter garbage data, we get garbage data out. It's essential to explore and examine the data sources that our cognitive processes use; in this case, our core and intermediate beliefs.

Let's begin by examining a situation that evoked fear or anxiety. What thoughts occurred in the moment that led to avoidance or other compensatory ways of dealing with the challenging situation? Ask yourself: "How did my thought shape my actions?"

Remember, your thoughts do not define you as a person. Your thoughts are neither good nor bad; they are not all-or-nothing. Your thoughts, irrespective of what they are, do not imply that you are good or bad. Thoughts are not pathology. Thoughts are fleeting and momentary, but they can create a storm in a teacup if left to their own devices.

Let's explore what this means in more detail.

Just a Thought

The attention we attach to a thought can make it feel real. However, thoughts are subjective and influenced by our mental state. For example, a person who experiences anxiety will have thoughts influenced by anxiety. Subsequently, those thoughts will not be objective or legitimate. Applying this recognition will open up a world of opportunity.

In the space provided, write down a thought that seems factual or real. For example, "I'm a great driver." Rate your thought on a scale of 1 (absolutely false) to 10 (absolutely true) based on how factual the thought actually is.

1   2   3   4   5   6   7   8   9   10

Rate that same thought over the next two to five days. Come back to the ratings that you entered on the previous page, and pay attention to the potential differences in rating at different times. Does your score change in different moments?

....

....

....

Reduce the Power of the Thought

Even if you realize that you are not your thoughts, that doesn't necessarily stop you from feeling consumed by them. Your next mission is to generate empowering thoughts that help create distance between your disempowering or negative thoughts and your reaction to them.

Offer yourself an initial affirmation: "I am bigger than my thoughts. I am not my thoughts. I control the way I think."

Then shift the way you refer to your thoughts using the following structure: *I am having the thought that . . .* Here are some examples:

Disempowered thought: *I am constantly worrying.*

Empowered thought: *I am having the thought that I constantly worry.*

Disempowered thought: *I'm an impostor.*

Empowered thought: *I am having the thought that I'm an impostor.*

Now it's your turn:

Disempowered thought: ....

Empowered thought: ....

Disempowered thought: ....

Empowered thought: ....

Challenge the Thought

Socrates was an influential Greek philosopher whose go-to party trick was critical thinking. He developed a series of questions to help counteract or challenge the accuracy of a particular thought. Let's give it a try with some similar questions!

The next time you are struggling with a negative thought, ask yourself the following questions. Write your answers on the lines provided.

- What is the thought?

  ....

- What is the evidence that supports this thought?

  ....

- What is the evidence against this thought?

  ....

- Is there an alternative explanation or viewpoint?

  ....

  ....

- What is the effect of my belief that this thought is true?

  ....

- What could be the effect of changing my thinking?

  ....

  ....

- What guidance would I offer a good friend if they were experiencing this thought?

....

....

Thought Evaluation

Thought evaluation is another form of critical thinking that allows you to reflect on which thoughts are real and accurate. It essentially presents the question: How do you know that this thought is true?

Apply the following evaluation questions to the thought that you're experiencing. Write your answers in the space provided.

What is the thought that you're experiencing? Take time to be clear and concise about the nature of the thought.

....

....

Why is this thought occurring? Ask yourself why this thought might be significant and whether you agree with it.

....

....

What's in your blind spot? What, possibly, don't you see or recognize about this thought that could be important?

....

....

How do you know? Ask yourself where the information that forms this thought came from. Is it reliable and verifiable?

....

....

What if . . . ? What other considerations or possibilities are there for this thought?

....

....

Thought Detachment

Creating distance from your thoughts by envisioning yourself as an observer can help you resist being swept away by your thoughts. Try this mindfulness exercise to allow your thoughts to float away.

1. Imagine yourself at a music event. There's lots of noise and activity, and there are people everywhere. Some are focused on the music, and others are engaged in conversation. It might be hard to concentrate and enjoy what the band is playing because of all the commotion.

2. Step back and be an observer. Change your relationship to the situation in front of you. Allow all the movement and activity to pass you by. Let thoughts, ideas, opinions, judgments, and statements "flow" right past.

3. Now take a moment to apply this visual tool to your thoughts. Imagine your thoughts are the commotion of a concert. Step back from your thoughts. Observe them and allow them to flow past you.

    Were you able to distance yourself? How did it feel? Did it produce any new thoughts or perspectives?

....

....

Worry Time

Allocating "worry time," or time for deliberate worrying, is a tactic that encourages scheduling time to explore and challenge our negative thoughts–especially those that are future-focused.

Schedule your worry time. Allocate 15 to 30 minutes at the same time and place daily. Avoid scheduling worry time just before going to bed.

Externalize your worries. During your allocated worry time, write down all the things you've been concerned about that come to mind in a separate notebook. Getting them out of your head and down on paper can be extremely cathartic, and you might be surprised at what you discover.

Compartmentalize your worry time. If you find yourself worrying outside of your allocated worry time, remind yourself to let those thoughts go until your next scheduled worry session. Observe concerns that pop up throughout the day, and practice catching them earlier and earlier.

Debrief & Digest

Well done, sir! Each chapter you successfully work through is an essential step toward finding calm. Even if you experience moments of discouragement, keep moving forward. A life without anxiety is just around the corner. Where you are is not where you need to hang out indefinitely.

Acknowledging the role that our thoughts play in interpreting and responding to the world around us is a vital step in reducing anxiety. In this chapter:

- We've come to understand that it's the meaning we assign to situations that arouses adverse reactions, rather than the situation itself.
- We considered the various cognitive distortions that we typically adopt and the impact that these thoughts create.
- We examined the construct that thoughts are just thoughts—simply mental events or part of a mental process.

Chapter Check-In

Let's reflect on what you've learned from this chapter. Please answer the following questions in the space provided.

- How do your thoughts influence you as a person?

....

....

....

....

- What form of distorted thinking do you adopt the most in your daily life?

....

....

....

....

- What additional information regarding the role of cognitive processes, or thinking, would help you in your journey?

....

....

....

....

CHAPTER 5

Conquering Fear of the Unknown

Intolerance of ambiguity is a main cause of anxiety. In this chapter, you'll discover why uncertainty can be so difficult. But don't worry—there are several tools and exercises you'll learn to help you manage these situations and make them less daunting.

You will also explore the significance of uncertainty in creating a meaningful life. We'll examine the correlation between perceiving the unknown and how the inability to remain flexible in uncertain times can create tension. I'll also go over the role of acceptance in reframing and navigating situations that you perceive as risky or threatening. Let's get started.

Dealing with the Unknown

Let's face it, the word *uncertainty* doesn't give anyone a warm, fuzzy feeling. People generally do not like vague or ambiguous situations, because dealing with the unknown is simply not comfortable. This is because our ability to avoid or mitigate undesirable consequences requires a degree of predictability—something that is not always possible to establish. Some individuals navigate ambiguous situations just fine, while others perceive them as threatening and respond with avoidance behaviors such as denial or withdrawal.

However, intolerance of ambiguity is completely normal. Intolerance of uncertainty is a human predisposition to perceive, interpret, and respond to ambiguous events as dangerous.

Put simply, ambiguity stems from new, complex, or contradicting situations. In these circumstances, there are complex factors to consider in reaching a resolution. These types of circumstances can make anyone feel uncertain about how to respond.

It's possible to increase our tolerance for ambiguity by changing how we perceive these situations. This can help us become more adaptable to change. But first, let's look at the creative ways in which the brain responds to ambiguity.

According to researchers, the human brain is an "anticipatory machine," and imagining the future is one of its core functions. When presented with a new and potentially threatening situation, the brain uses past experiences and knowledge to predict, avoid, or prepare for adversity.

However, when information is missing or questionable, the uncertainty diminishes how efficiently and effectively we can prepare. This irregular and excessive anticipatory response creates fear, a common feature in most anxiety-related disorders.

So what can we do to improve our response to these situations? Here are a few tips:

Remove the perception that ambiguity is a threat. We can navigate around the unknown by using something we all possess: our intuition. This is our sixth sense, or that instinct that guides you toward knowing that something feels right. Intuition is a scientifically recognized skill, so trust in this inner voice—it's providing you clues.

Take your time. Don't allow yourself to be rushed by today's fast-paced world into constantly thinking about what's to come. Practice mindfulness by staying in the moment. Anxiety is often caused by our inability to stay in the present moment and our propensity to dwell on the future. When we are anxious, we consume valuable mental and physical resources that are otherwise needed for effective problem-solving. Mindfulness is a valuable tool for slowing things down to free up these resources.

Learn more about the situation at hand. Request more information and do a risk assessment of the pros and cons of each path. Share your scenario with trusted others and request their input. The more information you gather, the clearer your decision will become.

Trust in yourself, step out of your comfort zone, let go, and move on. Realize that the best you can do is make the best decision with the information you have at the time.

Uncertainty is a very normal part of life. Ambiguous situations, although undesirable, are navigable. It's perfectly acceptable to temporarily relinquish control as we allow circumstances to take shape. It's also normal for life to feel messy sometimes. We're all a work in progress.

Meeting New People

Meeting new people can provoke social anxiety for a lot of men. Engaging with others is one of the most ambiguous situations we can face. In each interaction, there are many uncertain elements: determining whom to confide in and how best to express ourselves, assessing a person's trustworthiness, and establishing and respecting boundaries. This, combined with the lack of reliable, objective, and real-time information, heightens the brain's vigilance for impending danger.

The thought of being rejected or ridiculed can also evoke fear. Navigating these interactions is considered high stakes due to the significance that social and interpersonal relationships play in our well-being.

Starting a New Job

Men often convey that their work provides a significant amount of personal meaning. Traditionally, men derive self-esteem, gender identity, and happiness from their career. In some instances, it's more impactful than their home or social interactions.

This sense of purpose, challenge, structure, belonging, and ability to provide contributes to a sense of masculinity and self. When someone starts a new job, they are navigating a series of new and ambiguous social interactions and performance expectations. This can induce worry and panic about future social acceptance and meeting workplace expectations, as well as the anticipation of financial rewards.

Being Injured or Sick

For some individuals, the uncertainty of illness or injury can provoke a significant amount of fear and anxiety. The mind can easily become preoccupied with negative thoughts pertaining to one's competency, restricted abilities, the recovery process, and the fear of being a burden to others. The stigma associated with illness and injury often leads to a sense of vulnerability that men are fearful to present, as well as concerns about how others will view them.

Most of these thoughts are future-oriented and fall under the categories of catastrophizing (see page 54) or overgeneralization (see page 55).

Committing to a Relationship

Getting married, or even the thought of entering into a committed relationship, can arouse significant uncertainty. Committed relationships generally present certain uncertainties and risks, and we are naturally risk-averse and will avoid it whenever possible. Concerns over compatibility, the potential of lost investment if the relationship fails, the fear of feeling limited or that someone better suited could be out there, and the fear of being rejected all create an intolerance of uncertainty. Furthermore, the juxtaposition of the fear of intimacy and the fear of being alone can generate a lot of mental and emotional conflict.

Change in Financial State

A sudden or unexpected change in one's financial state can lead to an intolerance of ambiguity. The uncertainty of being able to meet financial responsibilities can evoke a deep sense of dread.

A man who experiences this is likely to be concerned about his ability to adapt to the change in his circumstances and how long the situation will last. He may also anticipate worst-case scenarios, such as not being able to provide for his family, having their utilities disconnected, or losing their home.

Financial situations are highly complex and influenced by a number of variables, and anxiety can make it difficult to identify solutions. Most licensed therapists can help with your emotional and psychological relationship with money if you're feeling overwhelmed. However, specialist help is available, such as credit or budgeting counselors or financial therapists, if mainstream therapy isn't sufficient. You don't need to navigate a change in financial state alone.

Competition and Conflict

Competition and conflict are a part of life, but both can leave many men feeling uneasy. For a lot of men, competition is essential, because men from a young age are taught that competitiveness is a healthy masculine trait and that they should seek it out. Competition is one of the primary ways men bond with other men, and healthy competition is a combination of cooperation and conflict. Men will often seek an adversary to compete against or an ally to collaborate with to achieve a challenging goal or pursuit.

For some men, competition can be very healthy. However, some competitive situations can be ambiguous and evoke fear and worry. Such situations may leave an individual feeling inadequate or worrying about the perceptions of others.

Some conflict is necessary in life, such as maintaining boundaries, speaking your truth, and standing up for yourself, but many individuals who experience anxiety will avoid conflict out of fear of how they will be perceived. This avoidance is not constructive and presents a host of other problems that are detrimental to mental and emotional well-being.

Recognizing Ambiguity

Start becoming familiar with the ambiguity that you may have faced in your life. Take a moment to reflect and answer the following questions.

* What thoughts, emotions, and behaviors do you adopt when faced with an unknown or novel situation that evokes worry and anxiety?

  ....

  ....

* What danger or threat might occur if you were to relinquish control over a particular situation in which you experienced anxiety? (For example, if you were to speak up even if you were afraid of being rejected or judged.)

  ....

  ....

- What does the phrase *acceptance without regret* mean to you?

_____

_____

Accepting the Unknown

Throughout history, humans have responded to the unknown with incredible creativity. From the moment we first gazed upon the moon in the night sky, we learned to increase our tolerance of the unknown by creating and assigning meaning to the things we didn't understand. Even in our contemporary lives, there continues to be a lot of uncertainty about the world around us and the unknown future in front of us. This can be disconcerting for anyone.

As we've discussed, it's a human condition to react to uncertainty and ambiguity. So how can we learn to successfully navigate and tolerate the great unknown of life as it unfolds with all the drama, complexity, and adversity of a soap opera on steroids?

What we can do is recognize that the scope of control we have over our lives is limited. Our circle of influence varies depending on the situation—and in a lot of situations, we overestimate our influence, which can lead to anxiety. Attempting to influence or maintain control in impossible situations often causes greater suffering than the situation itself, because it places an individual in a constant state of tension.

Another way to reduce anxiety is by reducing our circle of concern about the unknown. Reducing one's circle of concern is achieved through the practice of *radical acceptance*, or the recognition of reality—regardless of how it is experienced—without dispute, blame, judgment, or resistance. Adopting this construct allows a continuous flow of change that is accompanied by a sense of serenity. With radical acceptance, we allow things to be as they are and acknowledge that life sometimes consists of pain and disappointment. While pain is inevitable in life, suffering is not always necessary. When we reduce our attention on what we're trying to control, we can redirect valuable mental and physical energy toward things we actually do have influence over.

Similarly, personal acceptance is defined as *unconditional self-acceptance*. People can learn to accept themselves without conditions—warts and all—and develop a more satisfying and empowering relationship with themselves.

Acceptance in general represents a powerful first step toward internal change. It's not resignation or failure; it's simply acknowledging the truth and allowing certain things to be as they are. It allows for a deeper appreciation of life and more successful navigation of ambiguity, and it helps an individual flourish. The next few strategies will help you in navigating the ambiguous nature of the unknown.

Fighting the Unknown: The Pros and Cons

When faced with the unknown, it is common to experience confusion about which choices to make. A valuable tool in these situations is a decision matrix, which helps with examining the advantages and disadvantages of either accepting or contesting uncertainty in a structured and sequential way.

　　The main aim of this tool is to give equal attention to each option. Use this matrix when faced with an ambiguous situation to determine whether to accept or take on the situation. Write the various advantages or disadvantages for each option in its respective box.

DECISION OPTIONS: ACCEPT OR FIGHT THE UNKNOWN	
Advantages of Accepting the Unknown	Advantages of Fighting the Unknown
Disadvantages of Accepting the Unknown	Disadvantages of Fighting the Unknown

Once the advantages and disadvantages of each option have been identified, you'll reflect on the downside and upside of each. Identify which option you are willing to adopt and then, ideally, make a choice. Write down your choices in the boxes above, or replicate this matrix in a journal or notebook so that you can monitor your progress when examining other future decisions.

Sir, You're Probably Already Doing It!

It can come as a surprise for some guys that when they examine their life, they recognize examples where they are already successfully applying the tactic of acceptance.

Step back and reflect on all the possible domains of life where acceptance of the unknown or uncertainty is already working for you. Ask yourself how you think about these situations and what you do that allows you to successfully navigate the uncertainty.

For example, when someone cuts you off in traffic, you accept that there will always be dangerous drivers on the road. This allows you to be more aware of your surroundings, rather than be clouded by an emotional response. Another example might be accepting that layoffs at work are highly possible, even though things appear stable at the moment.

How can you apply what is currently working for you to other ambiguous situations that provoke anxiety?

Why Is the Unknown So Scary?

For some individuals, the prospect of a future that is unwritten and undefined, with infinite possibilities, is an extremely scary thought.

Write your answers to the following thought-provoking questions in the space provided.

- What is it about the unknown, either present- or future-focused, that elicits fear or worry?

- What situation or experience creates a current of anticipatory tension?

  ....

  ....

- Can you recall any ambiguous or confusing situations that you attempted to predict or prepare for and believed that you failed?

  ....

  ....

- What potential experiences, or lack thereof, influence your perception that something is scary or dangerous?

  ....

  ....

Take a look back and notice any successes, misses, and patterns of thinking and beliefs. It's easy to get stuck in mental patterns that aren't always accurate.

Life Would Be Incredibly Dull

Imagine that you've been anticipating seeing a new movie, and a friend blurts out the ending. You'd probably be upset, possibly angry, and disappointed, because you didn't get to enjoy the potential twists, turns, and excitement of what that experience would have offered.

If life did not contain any uncertainty, those moments of wonder and amazement would never be possible. The predictability of it all would be like a daily routine on a constant loop, like the experience of Bill Murray's character in the movie *Groundhog Day*.

It is important to experience uncertainty. In her 2017 TED Talk, psychologist Emily Esfahani Smith explains that moments of transcendence—those instances of awe and wonder when we least expect it—elevate us beyond ourselves and connect us to a sense of being that is considered a vital pillar of living a meaningful life.

Can you think of a time when you experienced unexpected awe or wonder? How did this unexpected or novel experience evolve you? How did it make you feel?

....

....

....

Embrace the Unknown

"Man cannot change the direction of the wind, but he can adjust the direction of his sails."

—Source unknown

This quote is etched on a paperweight that has been sitting on my desk for years. It's a humble reminder that there are simply things in this world that we don't have control over. It's how we regard the uncertainty that makes the difference.

Accepting the unknown is a bit like accepting the weather. A person can fight the weather, or they can accept and accommodate what occurs. Learning the skill of acceptance is being willing to adopt an open, receptive, flexible, and nonjudgmental posture concerning the moment-to-moment experience.

Willingness to experience whatever life presents allows an individual to move forward, rather than being stuck in the minutiae of the unknown. However, like any skill, there's a bit of training required to develop the flexibility and tolerance to successfully navigate ambiguity when it arises.

Modeling the Navigator

Can you think of anyone you know who is particularly good at navigating or embracing the unknown? What perspective do they hold about ambiguous situations? What language do they use to describe novel or uncertain situations they have never encountered before? How do they avoid excessive worrying? How do they willingly accept what is happening?

Invite them to share their experiences and their methods for dealing with negative thoughts or uncomfortable feelings that allow them to keep moving forward. What can you model to navigate uncertainty the next time it appears?

Embracing the Monster

Experiencing intolerance of the unknown is a bit like trying to go to sleep while imagining a scary monster under your bed. The sheer terror of peeking beyond the edge of the covers, fearful that something might jump out and devour you at any moment, certainly feels very real. The monster is fear, and your fear feeds the monster.

Allow yourself to experience the fear this monster elicits for a moment, without hiding, looking over the edge of the bed, or doing anything. Now give the monster a name, something nonthreatening and unassuming.

Imagine inviting this monster to a conversation where you share what frightens you and how it feels when you're afraid and anxious. Explain that it evokes uncertainty because the two of you haven't become properly acquainted yet. Tell the monster that you don't mind it living under the bed for the foreseeable future, and that it is likely that your relationship will change over time as you become more familiar with each other. Who knows? Maybe your monster will eventually get bored and find somewhere else to reside.

What thoughts and emotions does this exercise conjure? What does it feel like to invite the monster to stay?

Don't Fight the Riptide

This visualization exercise evokes thoughts of being swept away from the place you would rather be, and conveys that, rather than fighting the discomfort, sometimes it can be better to go with the flow.

Picture yourself at the beach on a hot summer day. The waves are rolling in, and everyone's swimming and surfing. You dive into the water—it's deliciously refreshing. Suddenly, a massive wave rolls over you and sweeps you off your feet. You can't feel the sand at the bottom.

You lift your head above the water to breathe and realize you're far from the shoreline, caught in a riptide. You try to swim toward the beach, but the current strengthens and you're tiring quickly. As your fear increases, a surfer paddles his way toward you, using the rip to travel with incredible velocity. You grab onto his board, and instead of fighting the current, you both travel toward deeper water. Soon, the water's flow eases and the surfer changes direction, moving diagonally to the beach. You are safe.

Your thoughts are the riptide. Don't fight them. Use them to your advantage and go with the flow. Navigate around them, then safely make your way back to shore.

What was it like to imagine struggling against the riptide? Does it evoke thoughts about how tiring it is to fight anxiety or the things you fear? Write down how this visualization made you feel or what emotions it brought up.

Changing Your Behavior

It's naturally challenging to create change that involves new ways of thinking, feeling, and behaving. It is very common to experience an increase in anxiety while doing so.

Some individuals notice that their anxiety occurs more frequently, or even more intensely, while all this heavy lifting is going on. That's why it's important to hang in there. This surge in anxiety is the brain registering that you're entering uncharted territory. The fact that you're detecting a discrepancy beyond your zone of tolerance is a prompt to change.

In the past, when you exceeded your zone of tolerance, you experienced anxiety. Now your brain is experiencing a significant amount of rewiring. Change that involves the development of new cognitive processes creates many new neurological pathways. It certainly feels like there's a lot of activity going on upstairs!

There's a lot of new information to digest. And putting it into practice takes time. Don't give up now—it won't be long until you start to see the rewards of all your efforts!

Debrief & Digest

What a monumental effort! Keep going to ensure anxiety doesn't stop you from achieving your dreams.

- We've explored key ideas, tools, and tactics to help you navigate ambiguity—a significant contributor to anxiety.
- We've recognized that intolerance of uncertainty is a very real human predisposition that everyone experiences.
- You've learned how to identify when you have exceeded your zone of tolerance and explored some of the practical tools to help navigate uncertainty—radical acceptance, unconditional self-acceptance, and embracing discomfort to lessen its impact.

You're investing in a life without anxiety. Take a moment to digest it all by completing the following exercise.

Chapter Check-In

Let's answer a couple of questions related to some of the key items in this chapter. It's always a valuable task to help reinforce the great work you've done so far.

- How would adopting acceptance help you navigate vague or unclear situations that evoke anxiety?

- If pain in life is inevitable and suffering is often an option, what could you do to improve your quality of life?

- How would life change positively if you were to embrace the uncertainty that presents itself in life?

CHAPTER 6

Handling Difficult Emotions

We now shift our focus toward learning to explore and manage unpleasant or negative emotions, rather than avoiding situations that evoke pain or fear.

We'll explore how avoidance maintains and exacerbates the negative cycle of anxiety and how you can break this cycle through a series of cognitive behavioral and mindfulness techniques. You'll also discover your own go-to avoidant strategies and consider what it would be like to accept anxiety rather than fight it.

And to help you stand your ground when feeling overwhelmed with emotions, you'll build a toolbox full of tips and strategies to aid you along the way.

When You Want to Run Away

Every one of us has a built-in desire to bolt when faced with situations or thoughts that are perceived as painful or uncomfortable. This coping mechanism is referred to as a *psychological avoidance response.*

Avoidance is a common coping strategy used to alleviate our experience of unpleasant thoughts or events. To avoid anticipated anxious or painful feelings that we associate with a certain thought, person, thing, or activity, we might try to create physical or cognitive distance from it.

This distance can be achieved by avoiding a situation, compartmentalizing or suppressing thoughts, procrastinating, suppressing a physical reaction, working long hours, and even engaging in substance abuse. However, even though some of these strategies are unhealthy, there is a valid reason they exist.

If avoidance didn't work on some level, we wouldn't find so many creative ways to keep doing it. One of the upsides is that avoidance offers temporary relief. For example, having a few glasses of wine at the end of a tough workday might take the edge off in the moment. Avoidance offers immediate and often potent relief of the unpleasant feelings of distress and discomfort. We feel in control of the stressor and the threat it represents, or we simply forget it for a while.

The downside of avoidance is that it is typically unsustainable, because it does not effectively target the underlying cause of the stressor. Avoidance may also play a crucial role in creating more stress and anxiety in the long run. Avoidance is a significant factor that differentiates people who have common psychological problems, like anxiety, from those who don't.

However, there is a tactic that can help with navigating the negative consequences of avoidance. This tactic is called *engagement coping*, and we'll explore it over the next few pages.

Identify Your Go-To Coping Strategies

Avoiding uncomfortable emotions may be considered a valid tactic in the short term; however, it has long-term ramifications. Without properly addressing avoidant behaviors, you run the risk of prolonging and even exacerbating the symptoms of anxiety.

It may not feel desirable to engage with the discomfort, but we'll explore a range of tools in this chapter that will help you achieve this. The first step is to develop awareness of the ways you try to numb or avoid pain, such as drinking heavily after a challenging day at work or minimizing or ignoring thoughts about a particular situation.

Here are definitions of the most common avoidant strategy types:

- **Situational avoidance:** leaving a social event early, avoiding arguments, being reluctant to walk in open spaces, not driving on the highway
- **Cognitive avoidance:** worrying, daydreaming, obsessive thinking, dissociation (disconnecting from sensory experiences, thoughts, and sense of self), negative self-talk
- **Protective avoidance:** procrastination, perfectionism, withdrawing, numbing
- **Somatic avoidance:** ignoring an illness, underestimating or overlooking physical symptoms, suppressing, or focusing extreme attention to physical symptoms
- **Substitutional avoidance:** abusing substances, self-medicating, engaging in risky behavior such as gambling, compulsive sex, or pornography use, or self-harming behaviors

Now let's apply these examples in the table on the following page. In each column, identify and write down five possible coping strategies. Use the coping strategy guide to gain clarity about which avoidant behaviors you use.

Reflect on your coping strategies as best as you can. If you struggle to think of examples, ask someone you trust about any coping behaviors they may have observed.

MY GO-TO COPING BEHAVIORS				
SITUATIONAL AVOIDANCE BEHAVIORS	COGNITIVE AVOIDANCE BEHAVIORS	PROTECTIVE AVOIDANCE BEHAVIORS	SOMATIC AVOIDANCE BEHAVIORS	SUBSTITUTIONAL AVOIDANCE BEHAVIORS
1				
2				
3				
4				
5				

Accept Your Anxiety

By actively pushing against or running away from unwanted feelings, you might find you are met with what seems like an equal and opposite force. The more you fight it, the stronger your opponent becomes. This is why acceptance can be an incredibly helpful way to relate to your anxiety.

Accepting that anxiety is a part of your life is not the same as resigning yourself to being powerless against it. Acceptance is not resignation, failure, or an agreement to accommodate anxiety. It's more like saying, "Oh hey, I see you over there, but I get to choose how I want to react to you and how much power I'm willing to let you have." In this way, you are able to receive the information your anxiety is trying to tell you and thank it for the warning before deciding what to do about it.

This state of acceptance becomes an active form of mindfulness. It is based on the belief that you willingly accept life's reality, including your experience of anxiety, without judgment, criticism, or resistance. When we accept ourselves, others, and life, we can develop a sense of peace and calm and minimize the suffering we might experience.

With acceptance comes an awareness, like when we introduced ourselves to the monster under the bed in chapter 5 (see page 81). This awareness allows you to confront anxiety and move through and beyond it. Moving through and beyond anxiety involves two steps:

1. **Practically adopt the practice of acceptance.** This is about changing the relationship you have with anxiety. A statement of acceptance might look like:

   I experience anxiety. I know what purpose anxiety serves. I know what anxiety looks like, and I choose not to fight or actively avoid it. I will experience anxiety in the future, and I am ready to receive it. In fact, I will acknowledge it and engage it when it occurs. This, too, will pass—as it has before.

2. **Remember that acceptance is not resignation.** Acceptance does not imply that you shouldn't attempt to remedy anxiety's impact. Engagement coping is a valid response, focusing on approaching the discomfort rather than avoiding it.

To engage with anxiety as it arises, you can turn to coping tools such as seeking emotional support, self-regulating your emotions, and using acceptance, cognitive restructuring (see page 60), or any of the other valuable tips and tactics you are learning in this workbook.

Invite Difficult Emotions

Living in a constant state of utopian bliss sounds pretty nice, and society often promotes happiness as our ultimate goal, but sometimes it's just not possible. As hard as it may be to accept, difficult emotions such as anger, disgust, sadness, and anxiety are essential elements in our human experience.

Instead of feeling bad about feeling bad and denying the way you truly feel, try inviting in difficult emotions and acknowledging them. I assure you, these emotions aren't vampires that will wreak havoc if you invite them across your threshold. Just receive these unpleasant visitors, allowing them to pay a visit. This allows you the opportunity to develop alternative ways of engaging them rather than being emotionally avoidant.

Bring Compassion to Your Emotions

When you remember that you are not your thoughts or emotions, it's easier to extend compassion to them like you would to any other visitor who dropped by. Being compassionate to your emotions is essentially about being self-compassionate. A lot of men struggle with this idea because of the stoic nature that our culture encourages men to adopt.

Being compassionate is about being nonjudgmental and noticing the disposition of the emotions that you have. Attempting to stuff your emotions down into the darkness may steel you against the moment, but this is the antithesis of self-compassion and will ultimately do more harm than good.

When you are compassionate with your emotions, you can navigate the more challenging ones and, at the same time, enhance your connection with yourself and others.

Sit in the Discomfort

One reason men are expert problem solvers is because they struggle to sit in the discomfort of undesirable emotions. Painful emotions can be just that—extremely painful—so it makes sense to attempt to resolve the issue, dismiss it, or avoid the situation altogether.

However, sitting in the discomfort can be a profound and compelling experience. Men often find this is hugely foreign territory for them, so they will adopt the most proficient survival skills available to remove, reduce, or avoid the uncomfortable experience.

Surrendering to discomfort means acknowledging the experience and just letting it sit with you for a short period. Start by acknowledging your discomfort and resist the urge to "fix" anything. During this period, you may find that you gain all sorts of critical insight and awareness.

Decode Your Emotions

You began this book as a detective, building awareness about the triggers of your anxiety, and now you get to practice some code cracking. Emotions are like Morse code, tapping out the various dots and dashes that make up our own internal messaging system. Avoiding or ignoring the signals means not being attuned to the message that's being received.

Difficult emotions are often providing information about problem areas, unresolved issues, and potential solutions. Taking time to decipher or decode the messages behind these emotions is essential to interpreting your experience. When you ignore or avoid an emotion, you miss out on gathering valuable information about the underlying problem. For example, irritation may convey the message that there is a personal need that is not being met. When you pay attention, it is always possible to learn something valuable. Emotions are a valuable source of knowledge and wisdom.

Recognize That Emotions Are Not Permanent

"This, too, shall pass" holds true for every single emotion. Although an emotion may be painful at the present moment, it is never permanent, though it may be hard to picture an end when the emotion is heightened or vicious. Emotions are not too dissimilar to ocean waves—they continuously ebb and flow against the shoreline. Each wave is uniquely different from the next, but once they recede, they are gone indefinitely.

Change is a central feature to life, and understanding change is central to navigating our emotions. No matter how intense a feeling may be, the next emotional experience is only moments away. You don't need to be run over by these waves of emotion, and you have the ability to recognize what you're feeling and choose which emotional state you'd like to foster.

Learning to Accept Anxiety

Take a moment to reflect on what you just read about accepting anxiety and how acceptance might allow you to objectively separate yourself from this intrusive experience. Answer the questions on the following page in the space provided.

- What would it be like to truly accept anxiety, regardless of the way it presents itself?

  ....

  ....

  ....

- How would you word your statement of acceptance?

  ....

  ....

  ....

- What would allow you to successfully sit with an uncomfortable emotion, without seeking a solution or answer to resolve the experience?

  ....

  ....

  ....

Stand Your Ground

Even at their best, avoidant behaviors only offer immediate and temporary relief from the intensity of unwanted emotions. Conversely, the techniques used with cognitive behavioral therapy (CBT) can lead to deeper, lasting changes. The specific aim of many CBT tools is to provide a methodical and structured way of breaking the cycle of avoidance, a core feature of anxiety.

Two components of CBT attributed to decreasing the fear and discomfort associated with anxiety are *exposure treatment* and *active coping*.

Exposure treatment is the most commonly used CBT-related tool in treating anxiety. Here, an individual is exposed to fear stimuli, either gradually or all at once, or by combining the fear stimuli with relaxation or alternative associations. Exposure treatment can help you feel calmer and more in control around things or situations you might normally find stressful. This tool also makes it less likely for you to practice avoidant behaviors.

Active coping involves actively choosing stress management tactics to control a situation that evokes stress or anxiety. This method teaches you how to adopt better behaviors and create new habits when responding to negative or fearful situations.

Through the use of these tools, you'll learn to react with more composure to feared objects and situations. By learning to create new associations with things that evoke fear, you can gain an improved ability to confront and cope with that fear.

Overwhelmed with Emotions

Being overwhelmed is more than just a stressful situation—it's a moment when you feel engulfed by negative emotions, like anger, confusion, frustration, sadness, and fear. It's common to feel paralyzed or want to run away from these feelings. For many men, being overwhelmed renders them unable to think or act rationally or even function. It's like someone else is at the control center of the mind and body.

Feeling overwhelmed is as uncomfortable as it is uncontrollable. The harder we push to escape or fight against it, the more the feelings persist. But with the right tools, you can find calm and balance. The next time you feel overwhelmed, try the following steps.

1. **Center yourself.** Now is the time to put your "break glass in case of an emergency" plan into action. Remember the CALM technique (see page 34)? This tactic helps regulate your emotions when you need real-time anxiety support. It allows you to reconnect with the rational parts of the brain, which help with controlling the flight-or-fight fear response, allowing you to bring everything back into proper perspective.

2. **Allow the emotions to pass.** Remembering that emotions aren't permanent is extremely helpful in allowing feelings of being overwhelmed to be experienced. Resist the temptation to fight it. Trying to control your emotions is like herding elephants. It's simply a pointless exercise. Allow these elephants (emotions) to go where they want. Then separate your emotions from your emotional response. You may not be able to control how you feel in the moment, but you can control how you respond. Feeling the emotion is not the same as reacting to it.

Running Away

It's instinctual to want to run away from feelings that evoke pain, fear, or discomfort. We know avoidance is a short-term coping method that offers interim relief and that it prolongs the underlying problem and exacerbates anxiety.

Engaging with difficult emotions is a positive coping strategy. You may feel you need to muster some courage initially to engage, so we introduce that first.

Mindfully create courage. Courage does not necessarily mean there is an absence of fear. Courage can mean that it's okay to be afraid of something and still choose to walk directly toward it. If you feel the urge to run, remember that if you run, you are likely to overestimate the danger and doubt your ability to work through it. Take a moment to imagine the thing, person, or situation—remember the paper tiger (see page 13)?

Envision a positive outcome. Imagination is a powerful gift, and we readily acknowledge that fear is our imagination running wild. Intentional visualization is a technique that encourages us to imagine how we'll feel after we work through the issue that we're actively avoiding. Imagine the positive outcomes when you are successful in overcoming the problem. Many professional athletes adopt a similar vision before a tournament or a race. They envision crossing the finish line or making that winning shot.

Avoiding Your Feelings

Emotional avoidance, also referred to as *emotional suppression*, is a go-to strategy for many men. Stuffing down emotions is a main reason why men adopt substitution coping strategies such as drinking, acting aggressively, or withdrawing. Here are several tips to help avoid suppressing an emotion in the thick of the moment.

Separate your thoughts from your emotions. Confusing what you *think* with how you *feel* is a way to avoid taking responsibility for your emotions. For example, you might think, "When my boss moves the project deadline without consulting me, I *feel* like I need to find another job." Recognize that this is actually a thought and not a feeling. Try restating this idea more accurately by referencing an emotion. For example, "When my boss moves the deadline of the project without consulting me, I *feel* angry and discouraged."

Label your emotions. There's a saying, "Name it, tame it." Expanding our vocabulary of emotions is an important step in expressing ourselves and thereby disempowering the impact of what's occurring in the moment. For example, by naming an emotion like "irritation," we externalize it. Externalizing an emotion gives us a better perspective of it, rather than personalizing it; thus, it's disempowered. For some men, this is like learning a new language and it takes time and practice. Refer to the Feelings Wheel listed in the Resources section (page 174) as a way to become more efficient at labeling what's going on.

Identify primary and secondary emotions. When emotions arise, it's common to pay attention and act on the emotion that is most dominant. For example, you might notice you're feeling angry but might not recognize that your anger is actually a secondary emotion. Another driving emotion, such as jealousy or shame, might be a primary emotion that sits beneath the surface. See page 2 for more on primary and secondary emotions.

Substance Abuse

Sadly, the most common way men try to deal with suffering involves alcohol and drug abuse and dependence. Recognizing when there is a desire to use a substance to cope with overwhelming or uncomfortable emotions is an important step in active coping.

If you are concerned about the negative use and impact of a substance, it is highly recommended to seek professional support. Seeking help for alcohol or substance dependency is not shameful and does not imply that you are weak; rather, it shows strength and courage. Instead of reaching for a fix, try these techniques to find calm in the moment.

Delay and distract. By delaying a behavioral response or reaction, it is possible to reduce the possibility of turning to a substance to cope. Constructive activities like writing, connecting with friends, or engaging with substance support networks are extremely effective behaviors that can help with overwhelming or negative emotions.

Find new meaning. It is often the meaning we assign to or the belief we have about a particular situation that leads to the need to cope. When faced with a challenge that makes you want to numb out with a substance, try examining the deeper level of what you believe this challenge means about you. Then you can consciously create a new meaning that can help cope with the negative or uncomfortable emotions that follow. For example, if someone expresses anger toward you, you might interpret it as "They don't love me, and I cannot imagine what I would do if they left." An alternative meaning might be "I don't know what's happening for this person; they could simply be hungry or tired."

Express Yourself

Emotional suppression—also referred to as the *prohibition of emotions*—is the main cause for many psychological and physical issues and disorders in men. The reluctance to share or express emotions not only restricts your ability to realize your full potential but also diminishes the quality of your connections with others.

It is unfortunate that men are not typically encouraged from a young age to express their emotions. Still, many men relish the opportunity to share when given the right opportunity. So how do you become more comfortable sharing your emotions? Remember:

You are the expert on your emotions. No one knows your emotions better than you. More important, no one can tell you how you feel. Your emotions are valid.

Put your emotions into writing before sharing. This helps you be clear and concise about what you want or need to share. Think of it as a practice run before you convey it verbally.

Be clear on your intention for sharing. Ask yourself why it's important to share your emotions. Understanding this intention can provide the willingness to share in the moment.

Create the right environment to share. Learn to proactively foster listening and sharing with others. When you do this, it models to others how you like to share and communicate, and you are more likely to feel heard and understood.

It is worth noting that sharing your emotions won't result in being engulfed into the event horizon of some massive black hole. Neither will it damage or alter your masculinity. It may be uncomfortable initially, but that feeling will quickly pass.

Debrief & Digest

Keep up the great work! Overcoming anxiety is most definitely hard work, and I have complete faith that you can do this. In this chapter:

- You learned that there is a built-in desire to escape or withdraw when faced with psychologically painful or uncomfortable situations.
- You were introduced to the construct of avoidance and how it maintains and exacerbates the negative cycle of anxiety.
- You've begun exploring your go-to avoidant strategies and considering what it would be like to accept anxiety, rather than fight it.
- You learned several tips and tactics to help you stand your ground when feeling overwhelmed with emotions.

Chapter Check-In

A mantra is a word, sound, or statement that is repeated to help with focus and concentration. Mantras reinforce and reframe ideas or intentions. The following is an example of a mantra accepting the experience of anxiety:

Acceptance is a conscious act of personal choice and power. The objective is to empower myself by disempowering anxiety. I do not "have" anxiety—anxiety is a state that I experience and nothing more.

Now create a mantra of your own that you feel will help you reframe your thoughts about anxiety. (You can also post this mantra in a place where you can refer to it often, like on your bathroom mirror or phone background.)

CHAPTER 7

Jumping Through Hurdles

This chapter will introduce you to a number of hurdles that most men learn to overcome as they tackle anxiety.

You'll become familiar with the role of procrastination and some tools that can help with this common form of avoidance. We'll also examine the behavior of worry and why this shapes the very foundation of anxiety.

Finally, we'll go over some basic information on the experience of panic attacks and how to prepare for them and prevent them from occurring.

Procrastination

Everyone procrastinates from time to time. Personally, I can think of about a million things that I've delayed over the years. Sometimes it's understandable to prioritize doing things we enjoy over things we don't. However, in this chapter, we're not referring to the behavior of putting off chores to go out with friends. We're looking at procrastination as an avoidant behavior that can be both a product of anxiety and the root cause of amplified anxiety.

While procrastination is a highly researched subject, there's no single description agreed upon to define this experience. According to the *Journal of Affective Disorders*, procrastination is referred to as an "individual's decision and associated behaviors of either intentionally, unintentionally or habitually postponing a task that is perceived as unpleasant or burdensome until a future time that leads to negative consequences."

The reasons individuals postpone tasks or responsibilities vary. Not all procrastination is intentional. Individuals who struggle with anxiety will often procrastinate as a way of unconsciously avoiding difficult or unwanted situations. Some see a task as difficult, not enjoyable, or something that requires great effort. Others will question whether there are any actual positive benefits associated with completing the task and will develop arguments supporting an opposing choice. Still others will state they don't know how to complete the task successfully or will spend significant time preparing or gathering information.

The dysfunctional nature of procrastination can lead to significant negative consequences. In the extreme, procrastination can be considered a highly persistent and emotionally distressing habit that can result in delaying basic responsibilities—for example, not attending to personal hygiene or other simple daily functioning tasks.

Constantly putting things off or trying to create a "work-around" makes it difficult to achieve one's full potential. Frequent procrastination diminishes academic and work performance, which then has a negative impact on mental health and interpersonal relationships.

The irony is that procrastination makes failure even more likely, consequently reinforcing one's ingrained fears about the situation. The experience of fear as it relates to failure is a key element of procrastination. Failure might be considered not meeting a desirable or intended objective or expectation, and depending on an individual's belief structure, this can be considered the antithesis of success.

Also ironically, those who find themselves stuck in this cycle may discover that procrastination prolongs and intensifies the experience of anxiety. It is not uncommon for cognitive distortions to occur; for example, you might feel bad about yourself for the inability to just knock out a task.

Whether you put off doing something because you feel anxious about it or you feel anxious because you avoided doing something, the link between procrastination and anxiety is real. As with other avoidant behaviors, bringing this pattern into your awareness is the first step in choosing different behaviors with more positive outcomes. Let's explore some valid reasons procrastination happens and what keeps it occurring.

Fear of Failure

Charlie has always been inspired by the idea of becoming a musician. He envisions himself being up on stage, performing in front of a live audience. After years of drum lessons, Charlie was invited to try out for a band that he admired. Despite the desire to pursue his dream, Charlie found himself delaying the audition, instead imagining overwhelming thoughts of freezing during a performance. His thoughts demanded utter proficiency, and he started to compare himself to successful musicians. Charlie visualized his friends and family teasing him for lacking talent. The thought of failing evoked so much dread that Charlie ultimately declined the offer to audition. He struggled to find the time to practice and eventually gave up on his dream.

Individuals like Charlie typically adopt the strategy of procrastination due to the fear of failure. This often leads to catastrophizing the outcomes and, subsequently, avoiding engagement in related tasks and activities to further avoid emotional pain. Addressing the fear of failure requires us to challenge the cognitive distortions associated with the meaning of failure. Here are three cognitive tools to try:

1. **Challenge your belief of failure.** The meaning we assign to failure can work against us if the belief is inherently distorted. How do you interpret failure? What lesson can you gain from failure? How would this alternative view of failure change your ability to engage in tasks and activities that you might otherwise avoid? How can you challenge and rewrite the old narrative of failure?

2. **Change your relationship with demands and expectations.** The demands and expectations we place on ourselves play a significant role in procrastination. If these demands are cognitive "absolutes," then failing can have significant negative consequences. Take a moment to consider the expectations and demands that you place on yourself. Would adjusting your expectations increase your likelihood to succeed?

....

3. **Acknowledge your resilience.** We frequently underestimate our abilities when faced with a challenge. Equally, we underestimate our ability to cope if we were to fail. How would you cope if your expectations were not met? What would it take to acknowledge your resilience and find ways to overcome this disruption to the path you chose? What does resilience really look like to you?

....

....

....

Weighed Down

Jose has been struggling with procrastination for as long as he can remember. At its worst, it feels like an overbearing weight. Despite his best efforts, the effects of procrastination slow down his life considerably. The gravity of not attending to his responsibilities plays on his mind a lot. He places a lot of pressure on himself to be more disciplined and organized. However, he finds that willpower only goes so far. When this happens, he calls himself lazy and weak. Subsequently, feelings of defeat creep in.

Jose's problem is not laziness or a lack of discipline. The real problem here is that he is stuck in a negative anxiety loop that perpetuates procrastination.

If you experience procrastination of any nature, ask yourself the following questions:

- On a scale of 1 to 10, how heavy does the thing that you are avoiding feel (with 10 being the heaviest)?

  1   2   3   4   5   6   7   8   9   10

- What thoughts are you assigning to your experience of procrastination? For example, "I'm undisciplined and I need to be better than this."

  ....

  ....

- What is it about the task that could be eliciting avoidance?

  ....

  ....

- What is one incremental thing you could do to relieve a small amount of weight you currently feel?

  ....

  ....

- What would it feel like to finally complete a first incremental step toward your goal?

  ....

  ....

Bad Habit

At the age of 16, Simon couldn't afford a car (he mostly wanted a Volkswagen Beetle, Type 1), so he ended up choosing to purchase a small 125cc motorcycle. He used to joke that his little Suzuki was actually a sewing machine on two wheels because you could hear him miles away. The only problem was he had to maintain it, and that meant that he had to divert money from more exciting activities. Even though Simon knew that maintenance was part of the agreement to keep the thing running, he found himself quickly developing the bad habit of jumping on his bike each day to revel in his newly found independence and freedom. He procrastinated, and eventually, one day, the engine died on him. He had neglected to keep the oil topped up.

You've probably figured out that this story is about me. And as you can see, even I can attest to the fact that habits can be nasty little creatures at times, particularly when the habits we've created begin to work against us. Many of the negative habits we adopt are related to some form of avoidance.

Procrastination is often a learned habit of evading or escaping. It's not always evident that an avoidant habit is being formed or employed. When the pain or discomfort of avoiding becomes far greater than its reward, that's when we often realize that it's time to consider an alternative strategy.

Answer the following questions to help gain a better understanding about the impact of unwanted habits.

- What habits can you identify that serve as a form of procrastination or avoidance for you?

- What are the rewards or benefits you experience by maintaining a particular habit?

- What are the potential consequences if this avoidance habit is maintained?

- What can you imagine the long-term picture to be if you were to success-fully overcome this habit?

Beat Procrastination

Procrastination is more than merely delaying a task or a decision; it also involves behavioral, cognitive, and emotional qualities. Overcoming procrastination can be achieved by adopting a CBT approach (see page 42) that focuses on mitigating dysfunctional thoughts and self-defeating behaviors. Here are simple yet effective cognitive and behavioral strategies to manage and overcome procrastination.

Make a Prioritization List

Having a clear understanding of what tasks need to be tackled is an important first step in overcoming procrastination. This helps you clear your mind of all the things that are less important so you can focus on completing the things that matter most.

Those who procrastinate often focus on tasks that are low in value, because of the emotional connection with things of greater significance. Tools like the Eisenhower Matrix (see the Resources section, page 174) can help you prioritize tasks by urgency and importance. Once the priorities are set, focus your time and effort on tasks that will yield actual results. I also recommend task management methods, such as the "Getting Things Done" method (see the Resources section, page 174).

Complete Quick Tasks First

Some tasks may be easy to simply "knock out" as they occur, rather than allowing them to accumulate or become overwhelming. This approach is ideal when smaller tasks present themselves that don't typically require a lot of time and energy.

You can also allocate a small amount of time for a task, like setting five minutes per task. Being mindful of how much time it takes allows you to develop a more realistic sense of time and energy that is required in the future.

Segment Your Time

We are less likely to overextend the amount of time spent on a task if a time frame has been applied. This is where time blocking comes in. When planning a task, think about when it will be done and how long that task will take to complete. Then, when undertaking that task, manage your time with tools like the Pomodoro technique (see the Resources section, page 174) or a timer. Having a self-imposed time frame can keep you focused.

Start Anywhere

Sometimes, simply starting a task regardless of the "ideal" starting point is valuable. All about creating momentum, this approach is helpful for individuals struggling with "planning procrastination," or spending an inordinate amount of time preparing and planning. Choose a part of the task that needs completion. Once you gain momentum, you're likely to remain focused. It's okay if you need to revise what you've completed or created—this is all part of the process of creating "flow." This method allows you to be more productive and not get bogged down with the thought that things need to be perfect.

Temper Your Expectations

When we set expectations that are too grandiose, or even too vague, the idea of completing a task can easily evoke procrastination. When you struggle with a task that is too big or complex, it prompts self-defeating thoughts about your ability to complete it and reinforces the belief that future tasks of a similar nature should be avoided. When you successfully complete a task that is realistic, you are more likely to approach these kinds of tasks with a positive mindset. This perception is vital in addressing the emotional fear commonly experienced with falling short of your own expectations.

Reward Yourself

Establishing a reward system for the successful completion of a task is an effective tool in overcoming procrastination. When we experience positive emotions after completing a challenging task, we are more inclined to approach similar tasks in the future with less avoidance.

Rewards work best when they are balanced on the nature and size of the activity. For example, allowing yourself to spend an hour watching Netflix after completing 10 minutes of housework may not be a proportional reward. Set contingencies that the task must be completed as planned and within the allocated time frame.

Adopt Routines

A structured daily routine that incorporates task management tools can be tremendously helpful for overcoming procrastination. To determine how best to structure your day, become acquainted with your biological clock, or "chronotype." A chronotype is the circadian rhythm that dictates our energy levels and ability to focus. By identifying your chronotype, you can create daily routines that align with when you have energy and focus. Therefore, it makes sense to do the hardest and most important tasks at the time of day you feel sharpest and most motivated. See the Resources section (page 174) for a link to a survey that can help you determine your chronotype.

Have an Accountability Partner

Personal performance has the tendency to improve when we "go public" with our intentions or plans. Sometimes the mere presence of others increases accountability. It's the difference between working out at home, where you might let yourself off the hook or take it easy, versus working out at the gym where you're surrounded and witnessed by other people pushing their own physical limits. Who are the people in your corner that you can ask to hold you accountable? Reach out to them and ask them for help to work through what you've been avoiding.

Offer Yourself Compassion

When you recognize that you are procrastinating, step back and offer yourself some compassion and self-forgiveness. This important exercise can reduce guilt and shame that perpetuates the anxiety cycle. Have a compassionate dialogue with yourself that frames procrastination in a way that acknowledges the purpose of avoidance. Rather than saying, "I'm a deadbeat for always failing to start things," it is more effective to say, "I recognize that I have been procrastinating, and I have an idea why I've been avoiding this particular task." By being kind and compassionate to yourself, you avoid negative thoughts that can cause procrastination.

Connect with the Bigger Picture

Remember your "why." By identifying the bigger picture or purpose of the task you're about to engage in, you reinforce the significance of why you're doing it and the future benefits you'll derive from it. This can help you break through the avoidance. Another effective tactic is to acknowledge the negative consequences of not completing the task. For example, it can be difficult to connect with why going to the gym today is important, but imagining yourself keeping up with the kids during summer holidays at the beach is a very real reason you pack up your gym gear and head off for a cardio session.

When you gain awareness about how and when you procrastinate, you can consider which of the tactics you just explored would be most valuable. Answer the following questions as they relate to procrastination.

- Does procrastination play a role in your life? What domains in your life are impacted? Consider social and intimate relationships, finances, career, personal growth, etc.

- Of the tactics we just explored to overcome procrastination, what would work for you? What have you perhaps tried in the past that you might like to try again?

- If you were to successfully conquer procrastination, what would life be like for you?

Worry

Occasional worry and anxiety are inevitable, especially when you're stressed out. Whether it's worrying about whether you have enough time in the day to get everything done or worrying about having a sensitive conversation with a loved one, intermittent worry serves a valuable purpose. In small doses, worry can bring your awareness to potential pitfalls ahead and help you prepare for the unexpected.

However, when worry becomes unruly or uncontrollable, it can be a real problem. Worry is at the heart of anxiety and at the foundation of other anxiety-related disorders. When individuals encounter worry that disrupts their daily life, it is likely that they are experiencing generalized anxiety disorder (GAD).

Worry is a procession of relatively uncontrollable negative thoughts and images connected to future outcomes. It is the processes of ongoing negative anticipation and the risk assessment used to prepare for, avoid, or solve an ambiguous threat and the associated consequences that we imagine might occur if the thing we're worrying about were to happen. Worrisome thoughts can shoot off in all sorts of directions, sometimes becoming more and more irrational. We can even compound multiple worries and envision increasingly unlikely catastrophic scenarios.

The act of worrying takes up a lot of mental real estate, especially when such thoughts become repetitive and obsessive. This diminishes the mental resources that we need to clearly assess and resolve problems and dilemmas that we might face. If worrying remains invasive, we are often restricted from seeing the possibilities in the world around us.

Excessive worrying can be pervasive in all aspects of a person's life. Because the experience of worry frequently leads to avoidance behavior, worry brings about anxiety. Worry-induced avoidance (see page 88) helps us cope temporarily. However, the underlying focus of our worry remains. This vicious cycle keeps someone who is struggling with anxiety stuck in the negative anxiety loop.

In some situations, anxiety-induced worry, left untreated, can lead to a wide array of cognitive, emotional, and physical symptoms. It is not uncommon for individuals who experience consistent and uncontrollable worry to experience panic attacks, depression, and even suicidal ideation.

It's time to dive into the world of worry by exploring some of the tactics that others have used to effectively halt this intrusive way of thinking.

Worth the Worry?

Martin is familiar with the rush of worry and the spike of anxiety that accompanies an ambiguous situation. However, he has learned several techniques that help him manage worry. To him, worry can be a valuable ally. He steps back from his thoughts and assesses potential scenarios and outcomes and the associated risks. He deliberates and reaches a conclusion about each dilemma he faces. He then declares to himself that any further worry is not beneficial.

This example highlights the fine line between constructive, deliberate worry and worry that is unproductive and relatively uncontrollable.

> Take a moment to think about a time when worrying may have served you and a time when it became problematic. What happened in each instance?

....

....

....

....

Worry Triggers

We all have an Achilles' heel when it comes to worry. Logan's worry trigger is whether he'll be able to provide for his family when his business goes quiet. His business is affected by seasonal changes, and he's learned over time that when business experiences a downturn, his worry is triggered. Logan knows that this one worry is his weakness and the source of his anxiety. Nothing much else worries or concerns him.

When the Greek hero Achilles was dipped into the river Styx to achieve immortality, his mother held him by his heel. This one spot was the trigger of his weakness. We all have an Achilles' heel—that thing in our life that triggers worry. Perhaps you worry about people you love, being able to pay bills, or a million other potential things that consume your thinking.

> Overcoming worry takes self-awareness of the things that evoke or trigger worry. Look inward. Look at your own triggers, and look at your life. What do you recognize?

....

....

....

The Stickiness of Worry

Everyone experiences worry in different ways. For Noah, worry has a degree of stickiness. Stickiness is described as the constant state of worry that doesn't leave and attaches itself to everything it comes into contact with. Noah describes his worry as one of those frustrating dreams where he finds himself running in place and unable to move forward. No matter how hard he tries, how much effort he pours into moving forward, there's no progress made.

Worry is a lot like running in place. It consumes a lot of mental energy; however, the very thing that consumes our thinking remains. As the worry cycle intensifies, you become more fatigued.

Take a moment to step back and reflect on your experience of worry. What does worry feel like for you?

The Worry Illusion

When Elijah discovered the real cause of his worry, he described it as a clever illusion. It was very confusing when he found himself caught in the grips of all his nonsensical thoughts. Not only did he find it disempowering, but it was incredibly deceptive. When Elijah worried, he found himself devoting a lot of his mental and physical energy to fighting his way out of it. He often found himself confused or stumped on what was the right path forward. It was like his attention was wholly misguided, just as if he were watching a magician perform an act. He eventually discovered that there was more to worry and anxiety than met the eye.

When you're caught in the thick of worrying, a lot of energy is spent trying to resolve a consequence generated by the imagination. Worry creates an illusion that there is no right answer to a problem. This is because worrying impedes problem-solving skills. To shatter the illusion of worry, ask yourself these three simple questions:

1. Is this actually a problem that I need to solve? If so, move to question 2.

2. Is this a solvable problem? If so, what's the solution? Write your answer below. If there's a solution, do you need to worry? If it's not a solvable problem, move to question 3.

---

3. Is this an unsolvable problem? If it is unsolvable, then it's time to apply the strategy of acceptance. For a refresher on the acceptance strategy, refer to page 76 in chapter 5.

Working Through Worry

Mindfulness exercises can help reduce experiences of intense worry. Mindfulness practices that include emotional regulation, cognitive restructuring, and emotional and cognitive expression are all valuable ways of working through worry. As such, you are proactively taking charge of creating an alternative experience and are no longer a passive participant when it comes to worry. Here are some practical mindfulness tools that you can use to empower yourself and overcome worry.

Move Away from Worry

This exercise of moving away from worrisome thoughts actually involves physical movement. The next time you find yourself caught in the negative worry process, focus on your body movement and breathing. By focusing on movement, you can interrupt the invasive and constant thoughts that consume you.

How you move is up to you—take a walk around the block, spend a few minutes stretching, or engage in more vigorous exercise. This movement can shift the focus away from your worry and help you feel more grounded. Incorporate some deep breathing, which will help you regulate your autonomic system to bring you back to a state of calm and presence.

Express Your Thoughts

This mindfulness practice involves talking to another person. I know a lot of men struggle with this. However, expressing your thoughts is key to reducing worry, because when you hold on to a mental image of a fearful situation, worry and anxiety stay with you. Expressing your thoughts verbally is an extremely powerful way to reduce negative thought cycles and consequential emotions. When you are able to hear yourself verbalize your thoughts, you're more effective at processing and understanding the underlying problem.

Also, articulating your thoughts, either out loud to yourself or in writing, reduces cognitive suppression. It is the suppression of thoughts that maintains worry and anxiety. When thoughts are expressed, you are no longer stuck in the negative thought cycle (see page 52).

Let's put this into practice. Think of someone you trust with whom you could safely and openly express your thoughts. This person could be a friend, a colleague, a family member, or even a trained professional. Preface the conversation by inviting them to just listen to what you have to share, and explain that there are no expectations for them to resolve a problem or present any solutions.

Examine Your Worries

Take a moment to write down everything you're worried about in a journal or notebook. When you document your thoughts, you can step back from them, knowing that your mind doesn't need to keep track of them. Think of this as an external complaints department that will record your worry for future investigation. Leave these documented worries in a drawer for a couple of days. Then return to what you wrote. Are you still worried about these things? If not, great! If you are, what possible solutions can you think of?

Disempower Worry

It can be empowering when you realize the paper tiger isn't that scary because it doesn't actually bite (see page 13). Start by reframing the thing you worry about by challenging the consequences should it actually happen. Rather than thinking, "What if (*worst case*) happens," change the beginning of the thought to, "So what if (*worst case*) happens?" For example, "*So what* if I make a mistake in my presentation?" The notion of "what if" creates and maintains worry. This "so what" reframe provides a way of circumventing the imagined catastrophe to connect with thoughts of coping and resilience.

Assess Your Worries

Step back for a moment to assess the role of worry in your life. When you recognize that worry is consuming you, or when it's acting like a silent unwanted houseguest, it's a good time to consider how to break the cycle. Answer the following questions:

- What mindfulness practices that would help you break the worry cycle would you be willing to try?

- What's your worrisome "Achilles' heel"; that is, what's your vulnerable spot that triggers your worry time and time again?

- What would it be like to express all the things that worry you, regardless of how big or small?

Panic Attacks

For those who have experienced a panic attack, it's not uncommon, amid all the physical symptoms, to focus on one distinct thought: *This is it. This is the end. I'm about to die.* Panic can evoke an unexpected and extreme sense of dread—especially during a longer-lasting panic attack. The physical symptoms may subside relatively quickly; however, the residual cognitive and emotional trauma can have a significant and lasting impact.

If you have never had a panic attack, reading the following sections could be worthwhile should you ever experience one. Knowledge of what occurs in the moment can drastically help lessen the symptoms and impact during and after.

Reading about panic attacks may be difficult for some, especially if you're familiar with the experience. You can continue to read on and learn more about what triggers panic attacks and how to prepare for them. Alternatively, you can jump ahead to the next chapter and continue your quest. There are plenty of other dragons to defeat.

A panic attack is frequently brought on by prolonged and unaddressed anxiety. Not everyone who struggles with anxiety will experience a panic attack. However, when a panic attack does occur, you may experience a sudden episode of intense fear that triggers severe physical reactions, even when there is no real danger or obvious cause. This can be very frightening, especially because it may feel like you're losing control, having a heart attack, or even dying.

The fear of not knowing whether you'll suddenly and unexpectedly have another panic attack leads to ongoing anxiety. This can affect your thoughts, behavior, and ability to function in daily life.

Triggers

Several factors may contribute to panic attacks, including environment, psychology, development, and genetics. Panic disorders are often linked to genetics, temperament, childhood adversity, life stress, and neurological factors. The experience is different for every person, but all panic attacks fall within one of three panic-related domains: unexpected panic attack (no obvious situational trigger or external stimuli), situationally bound attack (caused by external triggers such as a phobia), and situationally predisposed attack (panic that does not occur in all situations).

Physical Manifestation

Physical symptoms during a panic attack can include any of the following:

- Shortness of breath
- Chest pain or discomfort
- Choking or smothering sensations
- Heart palpitations (accelerated heart rate)
- Shaking or trembling
- Sweating
- Tingling
- Nausea or abdominal distress
- Dizziness, lightheadedness
- Feeling unsteady or faint

Psychological Manifestation

Panic attacks are often characterized by:

- Intense apprehension, fearfulness, or terror
- A fear of impending death or disaster, even though there is no concrete danger
- A fear of "going crazy" or losing control
- Feeling detached from oneself
- Feeling out of touch with reality

Know Your Panic

Now that you have a better understanding of what a panic attack looks like and what might trigger one, take a moment to reflect on whether you have ever experienced a panic attack. If you recognize any of the symptoms we just explored, please reflect on and answer the following questions.

- What was happening in your life around the time that you experienced panic?

  ....

  ....

- What thoughts did you have during the panic attack?

  ....

  ....

- What physical symptoms or sensations can you recall experiencing?

  ....

  ....

- What thoughts do you have regarding the potential of having a future panic attack?

....

....

Preventing and Coping with Panic Attacks

The following therapeutic and lifestyle tools can help decrease the potential of experiencing a panic attack and help you respond effectively if one were to occur. Having these tactics ready will help you feel less fearful and resistant during an attack and will make it easier to navigate your way back to calm.

Education and awareness. Men often say they mistook a panic attack for a heart attack and found themselves responding to it incorrectly. It's important to understand the causes and symptoms of a panic attack, as you have done here. Using the information and tools in this section, it's possible to reduce the potential of experiencing future attacks, and if one does occur, you'll be able to respond in a better way.

Acceptance. You can adjust your mindset to accept panic in whichever form it presents itself and acknowledge it as undesirable and not dangerous. Also, accepting the likelihood that a panic attack can happen again and accepting the symptoms when they do occur, rather than resisting them, is a powerful step to overcoming them.

Physical exercise. Physical exercise can increase mood-improving endorphin levels. These hormones aid in reducing stress, a contributing factor to panic attacks. Regular exercise is good for prevention, but try to avoid strenuous workouts while experiencing a panic attack. Instead, try light stretching or walking, along with deep breathing.

Meditation. A regular meditation practice can be beneficial in reducing the overall likelihood of panic attacks. Meditating teaches you how to slow your thought process and create clarity, both of which are valuable in reducing the cognitive activity that frequently leads to panic. Meditation is also effective in creating the ideal environment for adopting visualization techniques, breathing practices, and progressive muscle relaxation (see page 153).

Support groups. While many men experience panic attacks, few actually talk about it. This form of avoidance feeds the anxiety that fosters panic. Conversely, engaging in a support group allows you to release the burden and understand you are not alone in this experience. Talking it through with a trusted friend can also help relieve the burden.

But what can you do when you're actually experiencing a panic attack? Here are a few tips to help:

Acknowledge and accept. First and foremost, don't tell yourself not to panic—this will only prolong it. Accept that you are having a panic attack and allow it to pass. While you may be experiencing a tremendous amount of dread and fear and your mind is transporting you to that place of impending doom, *you are not in danger*. Acknowledge that you are not your thoughts, and this moment will soon pass.

Breathe. Slow, deep breathing disrupts the panic cycle and calms the autonomic nervous system. This may be difficult to do when you're panicking, but don't give up. If you have already practiced mindfulness breathing, you may find it easier to employ. The box breathing method is simple to use and highly effective. Simply inhale to a count of 4, hold for a count of 4, exhale for a count of 4, and then hold for a count of 4. Repeat at least 5 to 6 times. You'll find additional breathing exercises on page 152.

Shift and focus. Bring your attention back to the present moment. Look around and focus your attention on an object close to you. Engage your senses to shift and refocus your mind away from the negative, dysfunctional thoughts that maintain the panic cycle. What sounds or noises can you direct your thoughts toward? What smells or scents are predominant? What can you touch or feel with your hands that will command your attention?

Relax your muscles. Progressive muscle relaxation (PMR) is effective in reducing anxiety. It involves decreasing the tension throughout your body while reducing negative thoughts. PMR requires some practice prior to a panic attack for optimal effect. To practice PMR, tighten and release sections of muscles throughout the body in a slow and deliberate manner. When this alternate muscle pattern happens, it focuses attention away from panic and releases physical tension. See page 153 for a more detailed PMR exercise.

What's Your Panic Plan?

There are many options available to reduce the potential of experiencing a panic attack or more effectively respond when it happens. Consider the tools we just explored, and answer the following questions.

- If you have experienced a panic attack, did you find yourself adopting any of the tools discussed? If so, which?

- Would you change or alter any of these tools to help you navigate a potential future attack?

- If you haven't tried these yet, what preventive measures or tools do you feel would be most valuable to you if you were to adopt them?

Debrief & Digest

There is a lot to consider during this journey in overcoming anxiety. I commend your courage in working through another important chapter. Well done!

- We discussed one of the prevalent forms of avoidance: procrastination.
- We explored the equally important role of worry and why it is the very foundation of anxiety.
- We examined the dreaded experience of panic attacks and how to prevent and prepare yourself for dealing with them, should they occur in the future.

Chapter Check-In

First, select which experience has the most impact on you from the options below. Then evaluate the degree to which this experience impacts you on a scale of 0 to 10 (0 is no impact, 10 is extreme impact). Finally, write down a tactic covered in this chapter that you would consider adopting in order to successfully overcome the experience that you prioritized.

Circle One: Procrastination   Worry   Panic Attack

Scale of Impact:

1   2   3   4   5   6   7   8   9   10

Act: What tactics would help you successfully overcome your issue of concern? List some options here:

....

....

....

....

CHAPTER 8

In Your Body

Not surprisingly, there is a significant relationship between anxiety and the body. In this chapter, you'll be introduced to the concept of the mind-body connection, something that is gaining greater recognition in all fields of science.

Becoming aware of the biological and physical responses to anxiety will reduce your experience of life on autopilot. Through this, you'll find that you're better able to connect with yourself physically, and this awareness will help reduce and lessen the severity of anxiety's impact.

When Anxiety Floods Your Body

Anxiety is more than sweaty hands or butterflies in your stomach. It also manifests in other physical symptoms, which can maintain and intensify the experience. When your body is physically reacting to your thoughts, it can be hard to remember that your thoughts aren't always true.

When anxiety is experienced over a prolonged period, it results in substantial physical consequences. Here are some common physical symptoms of anxiety that men experience:

Headaches and migraines: The tension experienced when anxiety is elevated can lead to a low-grade pressure headache or a full-blown migraine. Chronic headaches and migraines are often a symptom of an anxiety disorder, particularly generalized anxiety disorder. They also accompany obsessive-compulsive disorder (OCD) and panic disorder.

Lightheadedness and dizziness: During heightened anxiety, some people may experience lightheadedness or dizziness. Often, there is an internal sensation of motion or spinning. This symptom is caused by the brain's vestibular system, which is responsible for sensing body position and movement in our surroundings. The result is a sense of imbalance. The parts of the brain that are responsible for dizziness are activated when anxiety shows up.

Difficulty breathing: One of the most common experiences of anxiety is labored breathing and/or hyperventilation. Hyperventilation is described as rapid and deep breathing or over-breathing, and it may leave you feeling breathless. Due to the autonomic system increasing heart activity, there is a greater amount of oxygen being consumed by the body. Excessive breathing can reduce the carbon dioxide in your blood, which produces hyperventilation symptoms.

Racing heart and/or heart palpitations: A racing heart is a universal symptom of anxiety. This is because the sympathetic nervous system controls the heart rate, and the brain supports this action by activating the adrenal glands to release adrenaline. Simultaneously, receptors in the heart react by speeding up the heartbeat. The heart goes into overdrive to prepare to fight or flee a threat. Unfortunately, for those suffering from anxiety, this tends to add to their nervousness and level of anxiety.

Chest pain: Men will often recognize the symptoms of chest pain as a reaction to anxiety. This symptom, called non-cardiac chest pain, is a frequent reason that men seek emergency medical assistance, as many mistake it for a heart attack. Research shows a strong relationship between non-cardiac chest pain, anxiety, and other related mood disorders.

Sweating and cold extremities: When your sympathetic nervous system is activated, it affects the sweat glands all over your body. Cold extremities occur during the fight-or-flight response, due to the body diverting blood from the hands, feet, fingers, and toes to send to the heart and other main organs and the large muscle groups. Because blood is also rerouted from the stomach and sexual organs, it's common for someone experiencing chronic stress to experience nausea or a loss in appetite or libido.

Numbness: Individuals with anxiety tend to experience numbness, also described as pins and needles, in the hands, arms, legs, or feet. Similar to the experience of the cold extremities, the body redirects its resources—in this case, blood—away from the extremities to the more essential organs. Numbness is often experienced along with hyperventilation, where there is an excess of oxygen in the blood, causing a reduction in carbon dioxide. Carbon dioxide is responsible for helping transport oxygen throughout the body. Many of these symptoms—dizziness, headaches, and increased heart rate—can also be attributed to insufficient carbon dioxide.

Joint pain: Chronic pain, especially joint pain, is commonly associated with comorbid (multiple conditions at the same time) anxiety disorders. There's often a direct correlation between anxiety levels and joint pain. Regular physical activity can improve both the symptoms of joint pain and anxiety, but ironically, individuals who have anxiety regarding their joint pain will often limit their activities.

Muscle pain and tension: Being on a high state of alert for a prolonged period will cause fatigue. Anxiety tenses the muscles as part of the stress response. A common symptom of muscle pain and tension includes tightness in the neck, back, or shoulders, as well as in the jaw or stomach. Many individuals will describe issues with clenching and grinding teeth.

Male reproductive system and sexual desire: The male reproductive system is influenced by the nervous system. Chronic anxiety and stress increase the release of cortisol (commonly referred to as the stress hormone), which, over time, can affect testosterone production. This can negatively impact both the cardiovascular and the circulatory systems, as well as libido and erectile function, leading to impotence.

Sleep disturbance: One of the principal features of an anxiety-related disorder, in particular generalized anxiety disorder, is sleep disturbance. Sleep is a state in which restorative processes take place at all levels—without proper sleep, the body is unable to repair and restore itself, and this results in diminished functioning and other issues, including increased anxiety.

Physical Symptom Checklist

It can be extremely helpful to know the various physical symptoms of anxiety and other anxiety-related disorders. They can be difficult to identify and easily misdiagnosed for a medical illness.

The key is to identify these symptoms early, before they become severe or create further issues. Here is a list of common body-related symptoms associated with anxiety. Check the ones you identify with.

❑ Belching

❑ Bladder weakness or frequent urination

❑ Blushing

❑ Body temperature changes

❑ Breathing difficulties

❑ Butterflies in stomach

❑ Chest pain

❑ Choking sensation

❑ Cold hands or feet

❑ Cold sweats

❑ Cough

❑ Depersonalization or derealization

❑ Diarrhea

❑ Difficulty speaking

❑ Digestion issues

❑ Dizziness

❑ Dry mouth

❑ Easily startled or sensitive nerves

❑ Eczema

❑ Fatigue or tiredness

- ❏ Feeling ill
- ❏ Feelings of paralysis
- ❏ Fever
- ❏ Headaches
- ❏ Hearing problems
- ❏ Heart palpitations
- ❏ Hyperventilation
- ❏ Insomnia or drowsiness
- ❏ Irregular heartbeat
- ❏ Jelly legs
- ❏ Joint pain
- ❏ Kidney problems
- ❏ Lack of air
- ❏ Lightheadedness

- ❏ Low energy
- ❏ Muscle aches
- ❏ Muscle cramps
- ❏ Muscle spasms
- ❏ Muscle stiffness
- ❏ Muscle tension/ sore muscles
- ❏ Muscle twitching
- ❏ Muscle weakness
- ❏ Nausea
- ❏ Pins and needles
- ❏ Pounding or racing heart
- ❏ Rash
- ❏ Red blotches
- ❏ Ringing ears

→

❑ Sensitivity to sound	❑ Symptoms resembling a heart attack
❑ Shakiness or shaking	❑ Tense muscles
❑ Shallow breathing	❑ Tight throat
❑ Shortness of breath	❑ Tinnitus (ringing in ears)
❑ Skin color changes	❑ Tiredness
❑ Slow heart rate	❑ Trembling
❑ Stomach pains	❑ Vertigo
❑ Sweating	❑ Yawning

Once you have completed the rest of this chapter and have adopted body awareness practices, come back to this list and check off anything new that you identify.

The Mind-Body Connection

Scientific evidence reveals that the mind-body connection is inter-twined in both health and disease. Research has found psychological factors to be involved in many chronic disorders. Research also indicates that emotional, psychological, psychosocial, and behavioral strategies can be just as effective as many medical treatments.

It's clear that the body and the mind are symbiotic, meaning they have an interdependent relationship. How we treat our bodies will affect our state of mind, and our thoughts will directly impact our physical health. For example, acute stress is related to a compromised immune system, and research indicates that the body has tremendous difficulty adjusting to or accommodating prolonged stress. Emotional health can be affected by the impact of prolonged stress. The effects of stress coinciding with psychological depression or social disruption are always adverse.

Emotional health is composed of your overall feelings of well-ness, the quality of your relationships, your coping skills, and how you manage your feelings and stress. The body will react to stress, depres-sion, or anxiety with a variety of responses, including headaches, shortness of breath, sleep disruptions, and depression.

Mind-body practices are an effective solution to these adverse symptoms. These practices have become very popular in psychothera-peutic and behavior medicine interventions. Techniques include:

- Mindfulness
- Meditation
- Relaxation management
- Yoga and tai chi
- Lifestyle modifications
- Progressive muscle relaxation
- Breathwork

These techniques can gently guide the body toward increased well-being, health, and improved functioning.

Mindful Movement

Here's a simple mindfulness exercise that will help you develop body awareness to become more present with your body:

1. Find a time and a place where you feel comfortable and won't be disturbed. Set aside 10 to 15 minutes, or whatever time you can spare.

2. Close your eyes.

3. Begin at the top of your head and mentally scan your body for any physical sensations or discomfort. Include your shoulders, arms, hands, chest, back, hips, legs, and feet, focusing on each area for about 20 seconds.

4. If you encounter tension, don't resist. Instead, imagine the tension exiting your body. Breathe. Be aware of any feelings or thoughts and continue your scan. The goal is to raise awareness of how your body feels at this moment. Do not judge your sensations; just acknowledge them and move on.

It's entirely reasonable to think that this practice is a bit unusual. It may even evoke a sense of uneasiness or anxiety. Give it a try. Then try it again tomorrow. Engaging the discomfort is all part of overcoming anxiety. Also, don't worry if you fall asleep. With practice, you'll achieve focus and presence in the moment.

Cultivate Body Awareness

One of the main benefits associated with mind-body techniques is the ability to direct your focus inward to develop awareness of what is happening in the mind and body. Body awareness involves an intentional focus of internal body sensations. Focusing inward is also described as internal scanning, and it is a form of mindfulness practice. It's much like establishing a dialogue with your physical self. The practice allows you to explore, in real time, the various parts of your body and any physical sensations you may be unknowingly experiencing due to anxiety.

Here are some benefits of practicing internal scanning:

It quiets the mind. Taking time to focus internally on the body and its physical sensations makes positive changes within the brain. It molds new brain pathways that are involved in managing stress, focus and attention, memory, and mood. Internal scanning, when adopted over a period of time, quiets the default mode network (DMN). The DMN is a system within the brain that, in ideal conditions, goes online when we're resting and is useful in managing stress and encouraging creativity. However, the DMN works differently for individuals who struggle with anxiety. Rather than create calm, it increases negative cognitive function and mental chatter. Internal focus retrains the DMN to quieten the internal dialogue.

It provides awareness of your body's unique response to stress and anxiety. Developing awareness is typically the first and most valuable step in overcoming any type of obstacle. What's happening in the body is a method of communication about interrelated activity that may be happening, either cognitively, behaviorally, or physically. When you are able to identify the message that your body is conveying, that information can be used to determine the source of stress and/or anxiety, and you can assess how best to address the cause of the problem.

It shows you where you are most tense. Most individuals who experience anxiety can readily identify the areas of the body that carry tension. Turning inward allows you to determine the specific location and the intensity of those muscles and joints that carry the tension. It also allows you to identify other areas of the body that are subsequently impacted—for example, neck and jaw tension that results in headaches. Scanning for physical tension brings attention to the area affected, which can then be treated with breathwork, yoga, stretching, or massage.

It cultivates self-compassion for your body and its cues. The advantage of awareness is that there is no immediate need to problem-solve. This form of acceptance creates self-compassion and acknowledges that our bodies are amazing, interconnected machines, yet prone to unique issues and challenges, just like our minds. Self-compassion creates a positive view of how our physical self responds to anxiety and paves the way to more awareness of what is actually occurring in the body, rather than denying or avoiding the symptoms. Ultimately, self-compassion reduces stress and builds a strong foundation of resilience.

Breaking Autopilot

A lot of men describe that they feel like they are on autopilot and that their anxiety maintains this vague, monotonous state. There is little awareness of what's occurring in the present moment, and it's difficult to feel anything other than the anxiety. Much of what we do—how we behave and how we respond to particular situations—is automatic.

Being on anxious autopilot is a lot like driving a car from one location to another with your thoughts immersed in other things. When you finally arrive, you are horrified that you cannot recall anything about your trip. You don't recall making turns, stopping at lights, or passing any sights. This is a classic example of autopilot, and it shows how astonishing a lack of awareness and attention can be.

When we are overwhelmed with anxiety, our brain attempts to manage the stress and uncertainty by "zoning out" and switching over to autopilot. Autopilot is a form of avoidant coping, and it detracts from engaging the perceived threat. Autopilot mode creates an inability to focus and concentrate, and in its most extreme form, an individual who is completely overwhelmed might experience disassociation—a disconnection from the self.

Disengaging from autopilot mode is achieved through various forms of mindfulness practices. By increasing your body awareness, you can bring your focus into the present moment and connect with the physical nature of your body and its sensations.

Let's try a simple exercise of verbalizing a physical experience for the purpose of breaking away from autopilot and reconnecting with ourselves.

1. Begin by closing your eyes and identifying one physical sensation that presents itself to you. What can you identify? Do you recognize tension in your shoulders or an upset stomach? Is it tightness in your jaw, or do you feel the residue of the headache you had last night?

2. Take a moment to ask yourself, "If these sensations could communicate, what would they be saying?" How would the physical sensation you identified verbalize its purpose?

Debrief & Digest

I'm always impressed by the fortitude that I see in the gentlemen I work with, especially when it comes to addressing anxiety. Well done on getting to this point in the workbook—courage and grit have gotten you this far. Keep up the brilliant work!

In this chapter:

- You learned various physical symptoms that can be related to anxiety.
- We touched on how anxiety resides in the body, how the body reacts to anxiety, and what happens when anxiety floods the body.
- We explored the benefits of adopting body-awareness practices to manage anxiety and why the mind-body connection is gaining greater recognition within the scientific community.
- We looked at practical ways to overcome the experience of anxiety autopilot.

Chapter Check-In

When a vehicle is running rough, diagnostics can determine the cause. While the human body is an incredible piece of equipment, understanding what's happening "beneath the hood" sometimes requires identifying and decoding the message the body provides. Let's work on decoding what might be going on with you. Reflect and answer the following questions:

- What happens when anxiety floods your body?

  ....

  ....

- What symptoms of anxiety do you recognize since experiencing anxiety?

  ....

  ....

- Finally, which tool, such as cultivating body awareness or mindful movement (see page 132), would help you be more present?

  ....

  ....

CHAPTER 9

Meet Your Fears Head-On

Throughout this chapter, we'll consider how to intentionally engage your fears head-on, and how doing this is the antidote to anxiety.

We'll also explore the concepts of desensitization and habituation, their purpose and benefit, and the various approaches to these practices. You'll be introduced to one of the significant approaches to the treatment of anxiety: exposure therapy.

We'll discuss how to safely practice exposure and engagement on your own and how to successfully create thinking practices that enable you to face what you fear; I'll also go over some potential obstacles.

Desensitization Practice

Avoidant behaviors and negative thoughts can make your anxiety alarm more sensitive to certain triggers. This learned conditioning is called *sensitization*. Desensitization is the opposite—our brain is taught that something is not dangerous, through repeated experience.

Also known as *exposure therapy*, desensitization is a behavioral technique used to overcome the fear or trigger that provokes anxiety. Research shows that adopting specifically designed, systematic, repeated, and prolonged exposure to fear triggers leads to a rapid and sustained reduction in anxiety. Simply put, by exposing yourself to the thing you fear instead of avoiding it, you become desensitized to it over time. The trigger loses, or at least decreases, its power.

The goal of desensitization is to create new neural pathways so a trigger does not evoke the degree of fear that it once did and to establish beliefs that coping with the situation is possible. Let's explore a few key methods of desensitization that are used to overcome avoidance.

Gradual vs. Flooding

Gradual, or graded, exposure is a technique where the feared things are targeted in a sequential manner. The tool that is used for this approach is called an *exposure hierarchy* (see "Fear Hierarchy," page 139) that ranks your triggers according to their anticipated fear reaction. Imagine a ladder, which you start to ascend beginning from the bottom rung. You begin in a systematic way of engaging with minor stimuli and progress up through the hierarchy of more challenging stimuli. Higher-level exposures are not attempted until the individual is able to manage their fear response to lower-level stimuli.

Flooding is a more intense and immersive exposure technique, in which an individual engages the high-level anxiety-evoking stimuli from the onset. This practice is usually adopted only after the individual has developed a range of mindfulness and relaxation techniques, which assist with coping in real time. The purpose of flooding is to expose yourself to the stimuli for an extended period in a safe and controlled manner. Because fear is a time-limited response, you may experience a state of extreme anxiety, perhaps even panic, but eventually you experience habituation—a decrease in a cognitive and behavioral response—and anxiety declines.

In Vivo vs. Imaginal

In vivo means directly experiencing an anxiety-provoking situation or stimuli in real-world conditions. For example, someone with social anxiety may challenge themselves to attend a party and make as many new friends as possible. This experience allows the individual to practice engaging with the feared object or situation in an authentic and unsheltered way.

Imaginal, on the other hand, is the practice of confronting or engaging feared objects, situations, or activities using the imagination. Emotional imagery plays an important role in fear and anxiety. By repeatedly evoking the image of the stimuli, the intensity of the anxiety response is diminished. The practice of using virtual reality exposure therapy has gained traction in recent years, and preliminary data suggests that it can be quite effective. With this technique, a person is immersed in a virtual world that allows them to confront their fears without having to actually experience them.

Interoceptive

Interoceptive is a method that exposes someone suffering from a panic disorder to the physical sensations typically experienced before and during a panic attack (rather than to a feared object or situation). The physical symptoms associated with a threat are strategically induced, and the individual is encouraged to remain engaged with the physical sensations of fear.

The target of exposure can include thoughts, physical sensations, worry, or painful memories, using either imaginal or in vivo procedures. This method effectively treats a range of anxiety conditions including panic attacks and panic disorder, health anxiety, chronic pain, and chronic dizziness.

Fear Hierarchy

A fear hierarchy is essentially a ranked list of fears, such as objects and situations, that evoke anxiety.

When exposure to a less intense item at the bottom of the hierarchy leads to moderately reduced distress or increased tolerance, a person advances up the hierarchy to engage with more and more difficult exposures.

Making the Right Choice

Naturally, knowing which exposure or desensitizing practice to adopt can be confusing. The option that best suits your needs is determined by the nature of the stimuli and how long you have been avoiding it. Finding an option is very personal, because fear is an extremely subjective experience. Answer the questions on the next page in the space provided.

- What thoughts come up for you when you consider adopting one of the exposure or desensitizing practices described?

- Which practice would be better aligned to help you target the specific anxiety, panic, or fear you have experienced?

- Which approach would allow you to safely tolerate and overcome the fear that has held you back?

Facing fears takes courage and a bit of elbow grease, but the strength needed to face your fear is within you. It simply needs to be tapped into and channeled in the right direction, and you've gained some valuable research-backed tools for approaching this challenge in an effective way.

Why Exposure Therapy Works

Exposure therapy, or the repeated engagement of fear-provoking stimuli, is a foundation of cognitive behavioral therapy for anxiety disorders. As we've seen, exposure takes various forms, including some of the methods mentioned already.

By attempting to extinguish disproportionate fear responses that may have debilitating consequences, exposure therapy can positively impact the lives of those who suffer from conditions such as anxiety disorders.

Other approaches to exposure therapy may include habituation-based models. Habituation aims to prove to the individual that the stimuli they fear is not an actual threat. Habituation maintains that if exposure to an anxiety-provoking stimulus continues for long enough, fear will decline and, eventually, the likelihood of that stimuli-invoking anxiety in the future will decrease. When an individual is no longer triggered by the thing that once provoked fear, then habituation has occurred and the cycle of anxiety has been disrupted.

Safely Practicing Exposure

Engaging in situations or experiences that evoke anxiety and fear can be extremely challenging, even under the best of conditions. For some, exposure therapy can seem like the triathlon of therapeutic practices. It's challenging because all the safety behaviors and avoidant strategies that you may have developed over time have at least helped reduce anxiety up to a point. The thought of exposing yourself to the thing you fear appears completely counterintuitive.

Equally, for individuals who are eager to address their anxiety, it is important not to rush through this process. Accelerating it without the correct plan in place may diminish the potential positive outcomes and even create complications or exacerbate the anxiety.

Success with exposure therapy requires patience, courage, and consistency. By working slowly through the process, you'll ensure that you are prepared for the ups and downs commonly associated with engaging and inducing anxiety. It is also vital to have the right mindfulness and relaxation strategies in place to cope effectively.

If it all feels a bit overwhelming, seek professional help with establishing a treatment plan that includes exposure therapy. Exposure therapy is not recommended for those who are struggling with, or have been formally diagnosed with, severe mental illness, suicidal ideation, or self-harming behaviors.

The practice of desensitization is a bit like learning to ride a bicycle. Run (or ride) with me for a moment. If you had the opportunity to learn to ride a bicycle or skateboard as a kid, you've already successfully implemented desensitization. Try to recall what it was like the very first time you got up on two wheels—maybe you had training wheels, which is equally important. The main thing is, you most likely feared falling and hurting yourself. You were undoubtedly cautious. You tentatively jumped back on each time you stumbled, and you persevered. You developed skills that allowed you to become more competent over time.

In that experience, you were working toward a clear goal—finding your balance and trying to ride in a straight line without crashing into anything. Eventually, as you built up your courage, you realized that you could safely and independently ride down the road on your own. You picked up speed, gained dexterity, and began to focus more on your environment rather than the simple mechanics of riding a bike. At some point, it became second nature. You were no longer worried about falling off—and if you did, you knew that you'd recover and be zooming off on another magnificent adventure.

When we learn to master our fears, the potential of finding new and positive opportunities dramatically outweighs the experiences of avoidance and anxiety.

Reflect on a situation in your life where you have successfully overcome the fear and now experience something far more rewarding. Write down what you can recall. What did you do to overcome the fear?

....

....

....

....

Facing Your Fears

The most effective approach to reducing anxiety is not just facing your fears but busting right through them, to demonstrate once and for all that the very thing you have so creatively avoided for such a long time is simply a toothless paper tiger.

Engagement and exposure are the ultimate antidotes to anxiety. They are the antitheses of fear and avoidance. They represent the act of purposely leaning into the thing you are avoiding, even if you are afraid.

The purpose of courageously facing your fears is to prove that the threat or the worst-case scenario imagined is categorically invalid. As soon as you experience a "eureka" moment, your mind and body experience a positive and dramatic shift, with the realization that you're in control of your anxiety and that the life you envision is absolutely possible.

Working beyond the thing you feared allows you to see with crystal clarity what the various beliefs and thoughts that have been working against you are. As a result, there is often a significant paradigm shift in the way you view yourself, others, and the world around you. There is also a sense of empowerment, accomplishment, and self-efficacy, which you may find has a ripple effect into other domains of your life. There is something extremely valuable to learn when you face fear.

How to Face Your Fears

It's empowering to face our fears head-on, yet it's wise to have a plan before we do. For a lot of guys, having a plan calms the nerves and keeps the attention focused on the actions that will yield the preferred results.

1. Take a moment to document five **situations** that evoke anxiety for you in the table on the next page; for example, "Conveying disappointment to a friend that they let me down." Next to it, write what fear that situation evokes, such as, "If I share what's on my mind, they will reject me as a friend."

2. Next, rate the **degree of anxiety** that each fear evokes on a scale of 1 to 10 (10 being the highest level of anxiety).

3. **Document what action you would have to take** in order to engage and overcome that fear, such as, "To approach my friend and share my thoughts."

4. Then **rate the degree of importance** you place on working through that fear.

5. Finally, **prioritize** the different situations, and then consider putting this plan into action.

ANXIETY-EVOKING SITUATION	DEGREE OF ANXIETY EXPERIENCED (1 TO 10)	REQUIRED ACTION	DEGREE OF IMPORTANCE	PRIORITY (1 TO 5)

Where are you willing to start? What does engaging your fear look like? Take a moment to reflect and write your thoughts in the space provided.

Exposure Obstacles

No matter how proven a method of therapy is, the effectiveness of a particular approach depends on many variables. Exposure therapy is challenging because the very aim of it is to evoke discomfort. If discomfort is something you've been actively trying to avoid, then leaning into it on purpose will be challenging. These are learned behaviors that you're trying to "unlearn," and a lot of men admit that it can sometimes take a few attempts. It takes focus and a willingness to experience the discomfort of these situations in order to overcome them. The following are a few examples of obstacles guys can face when adopting exposure therapy.

Setting the goal too high. The process of confronting the things that evoke fear takes patience and practice. This is a marathon, not a sprint (unless you're trying the flooding technique on page 138). Setting your goal too high can be demoralizing. When you struggle to reduce anxiety because you've taken on too much too soon, the brain interprets this "failed attempt" as proof that exposure therapy doesn't work. This reinforces avoidant behaviors and leaves you stuck in the anxiety cycle. Like any form of habit creation, when you experience small incremental wins, the mind is encouraged to maintain its focus and endure the fear—an important skill when things become difficult.

When anxiety remains the same. There will be moments when you might feel disheartened. It's normal for anxiety to appear the same, if not worse, at least for a bit. No garden is made without getting dirty, as the old saying goes. When doing exposure therapy, it is normal for anxiety to remain the same for a period. This is because the mind is trying to revert to what it knows as familiar. The mind will attempt to resist the invitation to change. Exposure is a practice, meaning that it needs to become a habit, just like establishing any lifestyle change. When your anxiety appears to remain the same, it's time to apply Socratic thinking. Ask yourself: "Is feeling the same degree of anxiety proof that exposure therapy isn't working?" What conclusion did you reach?

When anxiety fails to subside. Think about the length of time that you employed all the various avoidant behaviors before you chose to challenge them. Some individuals have been using some of these avoidant behaviors for as long as they can recall. Anxiety is naturally going to take a while to subside. The brain is incredibly tactile, and establishing new neural pathways is a complex task. The aim of exposure therapy is to foster habituation. When habituation eventually occurs, the brain fails to respond to the thing that used to trigger fear—it is essentially so boring that the brain fails to register it. As a result, anxiety begins to subside.

Debrief & Digest

We've covered a lot in this chapter:

- You learned about the significance of desensitization and habituation to the things that are feared.
- We discussed how engaging in a structured and intentional way with an anxiety trigger creates new neural pathways in the brain, and these new pathways reduce the influence of cues that evoke anxiety, fear, and panic.
- You learned a number of exposure technique options and were invited to consider adopting one or more of these techniques as part of your journey to overcoming anxiety.

Chapter Check-In

What a monumental effort you've made to get this far! End this chapter on a strong note by answering the following questions about tackling your fears head-on.

- Of the various exposure techniques introduced in this chapter, which do you think would be best suited to helping you engage the anxiety triggers you've been avoiding?

- Are there any obstacles you can imagine that might make adopting exposure therapy difficult or challenging?

- To ensure you are able to safely adopt an exposure technique, what protective factors (such as mindfulness, relaxation, or additional support) might you need to put in place before you start?

CHAPTER 10

Find Your Calm

In this chapter, we'll explore how to best connect with the ulti-mate goal of finding your calm.

We will examine the foundation of relaxation and its tech-niques, including deep relaxation, progressive muscle relaxation, and visualization, to understand how they can dramatically help you navigate anxiety.

The value of personal writing or journaling will be intro-duced, as well as how putting pen to paper can calm the chatter in the mind. We will also discuss the importance of self-care, including sleep, nourishment, and exercise—areas that a lot of men struggle with.

Finally, we'll briefly address the use of psychotropic medica-tion, which are commonly used in the treatment of anxiety.

The Relaxation Approach

Relaxation therapy includes a range of tools and techniques that foster stress reduction. It's more than simply kicking back on the couch or soaking in a bath with a bunch of candles. Relaxation therapy aims to release tension in your body and ease your mind into a calm and peaceful state.

Relaxation therapy techniques include meditation, yoga, tai chi, progressive muscle relaxation, abdominal or diaphragmatic breathing, autogenic training (imagination of physical sensations), and cue-controlled relaxation.

Relaxation therapy became popular in Western medicine and psychology in the early 1920s. In 1929, American physician Edmund Jacobson published his book *Progressive Relaxation*, which introduced the process designed to rid the body of anxiety by progressively relaxing various muscle groups. However, many forms of relaxation therapy have origins in Eastern medical practices dating back thousands of years.

Relaxation interventions focus on changing physiological responses to anxiety with relaxing and stabilizing effects on the autonomic nervous system. By applying these stress-reduction techniques, it's possible to short-circuit the fight-or-flight response, lower blood pressure, relieve muscle tension, and control the heart rate.

Applied relaxation techniques aim to induce a relaxation response, a physiological state characterized by reduced stress in the body and a calmer mind. These techniques help break the cycle of tension and anxiety felt in both the mind and body and make it easier to maintain calm.

Learning to Relax

One of the fantastic things about applying relaxation therapy is that there aren't any fancy pieces of relaxation equipment required—you already have everything you need. Here are several proven and effective deep relaxation techniques for you to try.

Diaphragmatic Breathing

Diaphragmatic breathing involves fully engaging the stomach, abdominal muscles, and diaphragm. Here's how to do a basic diaphragmatic breathing technique:

1. Get into a comfortable position lying down.

2. Place your left hand in the middle of your upper chest.

3. Place your right hand on your stomach just above your diaphragm.

4. Inhale slowly through your nose, drawing the breath deep down toward your stomach. Your stomach should push upward against your hand while your chest remains still.

5. To exhale, tighten your abdominal muscles and let your stomach fall downward while exhaling. Your chest should remain still.

Practice this deep relaxation technique for 5 to 10 minutes, three to four times each day. As you become proficient in it, you can move to a seated or standing position. When breathing, keep your shoulders, head, neck, and jaw relaxed.

Prior to starting this exercise, rate your current degree of anxiety on a scale of 1 to 10 (10 being the greatest degree of anxiety). Make a mental note of this.

Once you have completed the relaxation exercise, rate your anxiety again using the same 1 to 10 scale. Did your anxiety rating increase, decrease, or stay the same? Reflect on how you feel in the space provided.

1   2   3   4   5   6   7   8   9   10

Progressive Muscle Relaxation

Progressive muscle relaxation (PMR) is the counterbalance of tensing or tightening various muscle groups with a releasing of the tension.

PMR's approach is to tense and relax the various muscle groups in the body, one section at a time, beginning with the feet and ending with the face, abdomen, and chest. Here's how it works:

1. Get into a comfortable seated or lying position, whichever you prefer.

2. Identify the muscles in your body that you want to focus on; for example, starting from your feet and working your way up the body.

3. Inhale deeply through your nose and tense the first muscle group hard—but not to the point of pain or cramping—for 4 to 10 seconds. Exhale, and promptly and completely relax the focus muscle group.

4. Relax for 10 seconds before focusing on the next muscle group. Mind-fully notice the difference in how the muscles feel before and after each tension/relaxation.

5. When done, bring yourself back into the present moment by observing your surroundings.

Practice this deep relaxation technique for 20 to 30 minutes per day. As you begin to adopt this exercise, attempt to tense and relax all of your muscle groups. As you become proficient, you can focus on individual muscle groups throughout the day.

Prior to starting this exercise, rate your current degree of anxiety on a scale of 1 to 10 (10 being the greatest degree of anxiety). Make a mental note of this.

Once you have completed the relaxation exercise, rate your anxiety again using the same 1 to 10 scale. Did your anxiety rating increase, decrease, or stay the same? Reflect on how you feel in the space provided.

1   2   3   4   5   6   7   8   9   10

Visualization and Guided Imagery

Visualization, or guided imagery, involves your imagination. Start by picturing a scene that evokes calm and peace: maybe a grassy field in the middle of a quiet forest, a tropical beach, or even a sunny bay window. Allow yourself to let go of tension and anxiety as you visit this place.

1. Get into a comfortable seated or lying position.

2. Close your eyes and slow your breath to a calming, relaxing rhythm.

3. Visualize a place where you feel calm and safe. Visualization works best if you incorporate as many sensory details as possible, so picture it as vividly as you can: What can you see, hear, smell, taste, and feel?

4. Notice yourself feeling calmer and more peaceful as you enter your vision more deeply.

5. When you are ready, gently open your eyes, coming back to the present.

Practice this technique for 10 to 15 minutes each day. You can also incorporate guided meditation or relaxing music to keep you focused and calm.

Prior to starting this exercise, rate your current degree of anxiety on a scale of 1 to 10 (10 being the greatest degree of anxiety). Make a mental note of this.

Once you have completed the relaxation exercise, rate your anxiety again using the same 1 to 10 scale. Did your anxiety rating increase, decrease, or stay the same? Reflect on how you feel in the space provided.

1   2   3   4   5   6   7   8   9   10

The Power of Writing

One technique I highly recommend to the men I work with is the practice of intentional journaling. Journaling is not the "dear diary" that you might envision. Writing can unlock inhibited emotions and give us a safe place to express ourselves, which reduces stress and improves well-being.

I was introduced to journaling almost 20 years ago when I was doing some personal therapy of my own (yes, even therapists have therapists). I had never done any journaling, and the whole experience was awkward to begin with. It was difficult to determine what the purpose was—other than being part of the "homework" assigned at the end of each session. As time and therapy progressed, my writing evolved from completely free-flowing to a more structured account of my thoughts, emotions, and behaviors.

The exercise of writing was extremely empowering. It enabled me to identify themes and patterns of avoidance and engagement. It also became a valuable tool to reflect on and navigate tricky moments in life by seeing words on paper. No longer were thoughts jumbled or incoherent. They were defined and concrete. Even now, I write almost daily, in the evening. It has become a cathartic personal practice that I can't imagine not doing.

Like any type of practice, it starts with a simple intention. Following are a couple of suggestions to get you started:

Pick up a pen and notebook. They don't have to be fancy.

Find a quiet, private spot to write and choose a time that consistently works for you, when you can look forward to sitting down and spilling out everything that's going on in your mind.

Write without judgment. Start writing whatever comes to mind. Don't be concerned about spelling, grammar, or punctuation or the occasional bit of colorful profanity. Write like no one will ever read it.

Focus on Yourself

Focusing on your well-being is all about establishing the foundational elements in life that foster a bright, clear mind, a healthy, functioning body, and a life that is meaningful and fulfilling.

Contrary to a belief shared by many men, focusing on yourself is not a selfish act. Being intentional about "keeping your axe sharp" so you can be present in life means you can show up for yourself and for others, which is as honorable as it is practical.

Here are several foundational self-care practices that can help you stay sharp, calm, and focused.

Sleep

Consistent, good-quality sleep is one of the most valuable foundational self-care practices we can foster. Poor sleep impacts how we function in every way. Unfortunately, the relationship between poor sleep and anxiety can result in a catch-22, as poor sleep leads to more anxiety and anxiety makes it difficult to get a good night's sleep. Here are a couple of suggestions to improve the quality of your sleep:

Prepare your environment for sleep. The cooler, quieter, and darker you can keep your bedroom, the greater chance you have of calming your mind and falling asleep. The body's circadian system (the sleep control center) responds to a decrease in temperature. That's why a warm bath or shower helps induce sleep: Your body and mind respond to a rapid decline in body temperature, activating your sleep cycle. All forms of artificial light, including blue light, suppress the secretion of melatonin, the hormone that influences circadian rhythms. Place electronic devices somewhere other than your bedroom.

Limit screen time before going to bed. Switch off all cell phones, tablets, laptops, and televisions at least one hour before bed. Reducing the busy cognitive activity that occurs when you're still responding to emails late into the evening is a good start to getting better sleep.

Limit caffeine and alcohol before bed. Limiting caffeine and alcohol is extremely helpful if you experience anxiety. Caffeine is a stimulant, and drinking too much of it or consuming it too late in the day can increase anxiety and inhibit sleep. Reduced alcohol use is also valuable to successfully manage anxiety. While alcohol may help you fall asleep, it adversely impacts the state of deep REM sleep, which is critical in mental rejuvenation, boosting memory, concentration, and learning.

What are a few things you can do to help you get better sleep? Write two or three ideas below.

....

....

....

Nourishment

Many of us think about healthy eating in terms of calorie counting or following a rigid diet, but the truth about building the kind of healthy brain function that leads to clear thinking and a functional body begins in the gut. Because there is a gut-brain connection, maintaining a healthy gut microbiome (an environment that supports the growth of good bacteria and suppresses the growth of harmful bacteria) supports a positive communication network between the central nervous system, the enteric nervous system, and the gut. Here are some ways to maintain a healthy gut-brain connection.

Reduce the consumption of processed food. Research has linked consuming processed, refined foods with psychological disorders, including depression and anxiety. To help prevent this, choose whole foods, or foods as close to their natural state as possible, and avoid foods that are highly refined—think of a potato instead of a potato chip.

Introduce food diversity. Consuming a variety of nourishing, healthy foods encourages microbial diversity and helps reduce pathogens such as viruses, bacteria, fungi, or parasites that cause disease. Microbial diversity means having a wide range of microbes and bacteria in our stomach/gut that support health and well-being. Frequently swapping out what we eat fosters a healthy gut-brain connection.

Reduce sugar intake. A diet heavy in refined sugars can impair brain function and worsen mental health symptoms. Research shows that higher sugar intake from sweet foods and beverages is associated with the increased likelihood of common mental disorders in men, including anxiety and depression. It is suspected that sugar can cause inflammation in the brain and can impact neurotransmitter activity, resulting in mood changes. Reducing your sugar intake is a valuable step in promoting wellness and well-being.

What are a few things you can do to help you get better nutrition? Write two or three ideas below.

....

....

....

Exercise

Exercise is a golden pillar of self-care and improved well-being. Research suggests that exercise can bring about many physiological changes, which result in improved mood state, higher self-esteem, and lower stress and anxiety levels. Exercise also provides a distraction from anxiety and positive feelings toward mastery and self-efficacy. Let's explore a couple of key exercise options.

Do anything. Just 20 to 40 minutes of exercise can improve anxiety and mood for several hours. Engage in any movement daily to enjoy these benefits, brought on by feel-good hormones, better blood and oxygen flow, and a general feeling of accomplishment. Whether you choose walking, running, weight lifting and stretching, or playing a sport, all types of exercise can help reduce anxiety.

Dig deep and get moving. Not in the mood to exercise? It may be because exercise itself is a stressor, but it's a good one! It forces your body to adapt to the demands placed on it, thus making you more resilient to stress over time. This type of controlled conditioning to stress is measured by a decrease in heart rate and blood pressure and an improvement in mood and anxiety symptoms.

What are a few things you can do to help you get better exercise? Write two or three ideas below.

....

....

....

Medication and Anxiety

For some individuals who struggle with persistent or debilitating anxiety, medication can be a legitimate and necessary part of a holistic approach to disrupt the anxiety cycle. Deciding whether to take medication for anxiety is a personal choice and one that should be made with professional guidance so you can make the most informed decision.

If you decide to take medication, include it as part of a holistic approach to treatment that incorporates psychotherapy support. Several commonly prescribed psychotropic medications used in the treatment of a diagnosed anxiety-related disorder are:

Escitalopram (Lexapro): This antidepressant belongs to a group of drugs called selective serotonin reuptake inhibitors (SSRIs). This type of drug is suspected to increase serotonin levels in the brain. Escitalopram is used to treat anxiety, particularly generalized anxiety disorder, and sleep-related disorders, including insomnia.

Fluoxetine (Prozac): Fluoxetine is also an SSRI antidepressant and helps those with depression, panic, anxiety, or obsessive-compulsive symptoms.

Sertraline (Zoloft): Sertraline is also an SSRI antidepressant. It is used in the treatment of major depressive disorder, post-traumatic stress disorder, panic disorder, and social anxiety disorder.

Lorazepam (Ativan): Lorazepam is a benzodiazepine. A benzodiazepine is a type of tranquilizer used for the treatment of anxiety, insomnia, or sleep difficulty due to anxiety or stress, and seizures.

While medication is a viable option for some, these descriptions are merely informational. As a licensed therapist, I am unable to recommend or prescribe any of the listed medications. If you would like more information on the various types, uses, and suitability of psychotropics, discuss the options with your primary care physician or physiatrist.

Debrief & Digest

Finding calm in the storm of anxiety can feel like the search for the holy grail. Even when we're in the thick of the storm and we stumble, there are always lessons to be learned. That's a big part of this workbook—standing back to observe the learning opportunity.

In this chapter:

- We explored the foundation of relaxation and its techniques, and how it can dramatically help you mitigate and overcome the effects of anxiety.
- You were introduced to some common relaxation options, including deep relaxation, progressive muscle relaxation, and visualization.
- We discussed the benefits of starting a personal journal to document your thoughts, emotions, and experiences.
- We introduced the importance of focusing on yourself in terms of self-care and the importance of sleep, nutrition, and exercise as tools to help reduce the impact of anxiety.

Chapter Check-In

Wonderful job getting to this place in the workbook! It's a monumental effort to dig in deep and to have done all this incredible work. It's a credit to you.

Before moving on to the next chapter, here are a few questions regarding the importance of relaxation and support in your life.

- How has anxiety potentially limited your ability to focus on your overall well-being, including nutrition, quality sleep, and exercise?

- Of the options presented in this chapter, what deep relaxation technique would you consider trying, and why?

  ....

  ....

  ....

  ....

- What are your thoughts on seeking medical support, particularly the integrated use of psychotropic medications, to help navigate anxiety?

  ....

  ....

  ....

  ....

CHAPTER 11

Choose Your Path

You're in the homestretch! This last chapter looks at bringing together all the tips, tools, and techniques you've been introduced to throughout this workbook and incorporating them into an effective plan.

An ongoing practice for yourself is the key to successfully overcoming anxiety and finding your calm. Any form of practice involves translating knowledge into application. This is where the rubber hits the road, gentlemen.

Define Your Growth

Anxiety is part of the human condition. It will always exist, showing up throughout life in various shapes and forms, and to an extent, it serves a valuable purpose.

It's only when anxiety goes unchecked that it takes on a life of its own and feels threatening or overwhelming. It may seem like anxiety is an intrusive, disruptive, and even tormenting houseguest that never leaves. However, no matter how long this unpleasant experience has taken up residence in your life, you can make the choice to show it the door.

When you choose to face your anxiety, you make the decision to face the paper tigers that have filled your mind with fear and uncertainty. By realizing that anxiety is simply comprised of anticipated or imaginary fear, you'll find that, with practice, you're able to catch your unpleasant thoughts, emotions, or physical reactions in time to disarm them before they carry you away. When you do this, you'll find anxiety loses its influence over you.

Don't let anxiety trick you into underestimating your abilities. You might be surprised to discover that living with anxiety has already helped you develop a range of skills, including resilience and fortitude. You are a fighter!

A lot of men who are triumphant in overcoming anxiety share that they were surprised at how much anxiety permeated into other areas of their world—and how challenging anxiety opened up their mind to what is truly important to them.

You get to define your growth. And you get to define the possibilities of your life.

How Will You Define Your Path?

Let's take a moment to define what life would be like without the heavy burden of anxiety. Answer the following questions in the space provided.

- How will you apply the knowledge or experience you have acquired to anxiety? What will help you overcome it?

....

....

....

- What areas of your life will change or improve when you are successful in addressing the impact and influence of anxiety?

....

....

....

- What untapped potential or opportunities might you discover when anxiety has been effectively confronted?

....

....

....

Target Anxiety Challenges

There's really no such thing as a foolproof anxiety plan. It's entirely possible that the unwanted houseguest of anxiety will present itself once again. Anxiety has the ability to evolve with incredible stealth.

Managing and navigating anxiety is all about the practice. Regardless of the level of mastery or proficiency you acquire over anxiety, you will always be an avid student. A best-practice approach to anxiety is to effectively prepare for when it recurs. The following are some suggestions on how to best prepare.

Understand Your Anxiety

Your experience of anxiety is highly subjective and unique. This workbook has focused on the importance of truly understanding your experience of anxiety. Knowledge of the various triggers, thoughts, emotions, behaviors, and symptoms associated with your experience is highly valuable. A thorough understanding of these elements will allow you to recognize if and when anxiety recurs. Know the signs and be prepared.

Know What Works for You

You are the expert on you. This simple notion can help you determine what best supports your needs and vision of overcoming anxiety. With this in mind, take time to try the various tools and techniques outlined in this workbook. Take with you what works and discard those things that don't. It may require some tailoring. In the end, it may not be the precise combination of techniques that makes a difference, but the very fact that you maintain them as an ongoing practice that gives you the edge.

Create a Plan

Take some time to sit down and draft a personalized plan for managing the challenges you face. Create a goal or vision for yourself and include outcomes that you hope to experience. Include the tools that you want to adopt as part of your "anxiety toolkit." Detail when these tools are to be used and for what purpose. Include specific tactics for what you will do if or when anxiety arises unexpectedly. Consider your life from a holistic, 40,000-foot view and incorporate any lifestyle changes you think might prevent the onset of anxiety. Most important, write down as part of this plan how you will celebrate your success.

Strategies for Growth

Just like your body requires certain things to maintain its health, your mental health also needs constant attention. Maintaining your mental health involves practicing self-care, adopting awareness techniques and coping strategies, and knowing when to seek professional help. Intentional upkeep helps maintain good health and prevent unnecessary decline. Continued attention to your mental health is also a significant part of keeping anxiety at bay once it has decreased in intensity and duration. Your customized maintenance plan should bring together all the tools and tactics in a succinct way that you can refer to on an ongoing basis.

Envision Growth

Let's begin with the long game in mind. An ideal starting point: Document your immediate, intermediate, and long-term hopes and intentions to reduce the frequency and intensity of anxiety. Spend some time envisioning what the improvements in your quality of life and well-being will be and add these to your plan. What lifestyle changes do you expect over the next couple of years, or even the next 10 years? By thinking this far out, you expand the vision of the possibilities and reduce the pressure to do everything right away.

Continued Self-Assessment

As part of your maintenance plan, reflect on how you will continue to monitor the various triggers and warning signs or symptoms of anxiety. Reflect on what you can introduce into your life to protect you in the long run. Document the various triggers and symptoms you've become aware of. You now know that triggers and symptoms are key indicators that something important is out of alignment and that it's time to activate an appropriate response.

Harness Ambiguity

You've changed your relationship with ambiguity. This will be an important factor in maintaining the great work you've done. Engaging ambiguity rather than avoiding it is both a mindset and a practice. You'll want to continue challenging your interpretation of what presents itself as ambiguous—leaning into the uncertain is extremely valuable in developing resilience. Take time to reflect on the alternative ways you can look at the unfamiliar and lean into it by asking what lesson you can take from the experience. Know that despite the circumstances, there is always something to learn.

Develop Your Knowledge

Keep learning about anxiety as part of your maintenance plan. While this workbook offers a fair amount of information, it only scratches the surface of what we know about anxiety. Knowledge is empowering, and by deepening your understanding of your experience of anxiety, you can navigate it more effectively. For many people, anxiety isn't caused by one specific thing or some cataclysmic event. It is often a culmination of subtle and unique things that roll up into a perfect storm. Knowledge of how the weather works helps us determine if we need an umbrella or sunscreen.

Self-Care Practices

Few men profess to dislike self-care once they become familiar with the practice. While it may take some getting used to, self-care is crucial to any maintenance plan for managing anxiety and the cornerstone of reducing the onset of any mental health issue. The foundations of self-care include a healthy diet, exercise, socialization, good-quality sleep (this is a big one), pursuit of personal interests, reducing significant stressors, and fostering calm. Take some time to plan out these rewarding elements and consider how you could incorporate them into your lifestyle over the long term.

Anxiety Adversity Management

Even with the best of intentions, anxiety can catch you completely by surprise. Plan a range of contingencies you can enlist when anxiety strikes. Document what you'll do—which tools and support you'll kick into action to help diffuse your anxiety. For example, know what action steps you'd take if a panic attack were to occur suddenly. Identify whom you might share your coping and recovery plan with, and talk to them in advance, so you always have someone you trust and who understands.

Manage Disappointment and Perception of Failure

We all fall over and make mistakes from time to time. Men often have a tenuous relationship with failure and believe they are seen as weak or inadequate if things don't work as expected. These types of self-imposed demands can perpetuate anxiety. Take some time to document what you will think and do if you find yourself in the thick of anxiety once again. Ask yourself how you might actually grow from a perceived failure or setback and what could be different in the future.

Find Your Support

Consider this workbook just one of the many potential tools in your toolkit. It can help to consider additional options that, when combined, will enable you to successfully move forward and prosper. I've included many resources for additional support (see page 173), but generally speaking, here are some of the options available:

Online courses: There are a wide range of effective online courses and programs that focus on education and management of anxiety-related disorders. Many are affordable and can be accessed on demand, meaning you can participate at your convenience.

Support groups: In-person and virtual support groups provide the opportunity to share the experience of anxiety with others who can offer mutual guidance and empathy. They allow participants to collaborate on strategies to successfully navigate anxiety. Support groups are easily accessible, widely available, and often very affordable.

Individual psychotherapy: Sometimes, professional support is needed when a self-treatment approach doesn't appear to be working as expected. Individual psychotherapy, also referred to as talk therapy, is highly personalized and focuses on specific needs and issues. Individual psychotherapy is provided by a trained, licensed health care professional. It can be accessed, either in person or virtually, which is often referred to as telehealth services.

Forward Motion Is Still Progress

Many of the men I have the honor of working with overcome the heavy burden of anxiety. Some may have only struggled with anxiety for a short time, while others have known it their entire lives. When these men find the courage to seek change and do the work, the positive impact on their life can be profound. With the right support in their corner, these men discover that anything is possible, especially when they realize that anxiety does not need to dominate their life.

It is not uncommon for men to underestimate their abilities—anxiety has the tendency to make you feel defeated. Just thinking about taking on anxiety can provoke anxiety, yet when they realize that facing this opponent will help them reach their full potential, the world opens up to them.

You are an untapped reservoir of potential. By accessing and adopting the various tips, tools, and techniques outlined in this workbook, as well as the vast array of information and services at your disposal, you are well equipped to access your highest potential.

I commend your courage in facing anxiety and working to establish a practice to overcome anxiety and find your calm. It may not always be easy, but remember: You are resilient and capable, and now you are informed. Your choice to take this journey is testament to the innate power that resides within.

Resources

The following resources offer additional and supplementary help and assistance for anxiety-related concerns and issues.

Websites

Anxiety.org: Anxiety.org

Anxiety and Depression Association of America: ADAA.org

Anxiety Canada: AnxietyCanada.com

Anxiety Treatment Australia: AnxietyAustralia.com.au

Anxiety UK: AnxietyUK.org.uk

American Psychological Association: APA.org

Beck Institute for Cognitive Behavioral Therapy: BeckInstitute.org

Black Dog Institute: BlackDogInstitute.org.au

Calm Clinic: CalmClinic.com

National Alliance on Mental Illness: NAMI.org

National Institute of Mental Health: NIMH.NIH.gov

National Suicide Prevention Lifeline: SuicidePreventionLifeline.org

The Anxiety Network: AnxietyNetwork.com

Tools & Apps

Anxiety Reliever: AnxietyRelieverApp.com
An app that provides calming audio recordings, helpful guides, an insightful tracker, breathing tool, and supportive messages.

Automated Morningness-Eveningness Questionnaire: CET-Surveys.com/index
.php?sid=61524&newtest=Y&lang=en
A survey to determine your circadian rhythm types.

Calm: Calm.com
For meditation, sleep, and relaxation.

Happify: my.Happify.com
An app to overcome negative thoughts, stress, and life's challenges.

Headspace: Headspace.com
An app for mindfulness and meditation.

Pomodoro Technique: Todoist.com/productivity-methods/pomodoro-technique
A tool to help beat procrastination.

Sanvello: Sanvello.com
For mindfulness, mood, and health tracking.

WorryWatch: WorryWatch.com
An app to help you work through your worry.

Videos

Anxiety and Depression Association of America: ADAA.org/about-adaa/press-room
/multimedia/videos

TED. Emily Esfahani Smith (2017). "There's more to life than being happy":
TED.com/talks/emily_esfahani_smith_there_s_more_to_life_than_being_happy

TED. Olivia Remes (2019). "How to cope with anxiety": TED.com/talks/olivia
_remes_how_to_cope_with_anxiety

Additional Resources

Getting Things Done (GTD): GettingThingsDone.com

The Eisenhower Matrix: Eisenhower.me/eisenhower-matrix

The Feelings Wheel: FeelingsWheel.com

References

"About Mental Illness: Treatments." National Alliance on Mental Health. Accessed October 2020. nami.org/about-mental-illness/treatments.

Adcroft, Sean Kennedy. "Developing self-regulated learning with time management and mindfulness practice." Dissertation, Fordham University, 2018.

Allen, David. *Getting things done. The art of stress-free productivity*. New York: Penguin Books, 2002.

Al-Mosaiwi, Mohammed, and Tom Johnstone. "In an absolute state: Elevated use of absolutist words is a marker specific to anxiety, depression, and suicidal ideation." *Clinical Psychological Science* 6, no. 4 (January 2018): 529–542. doi:10.1177/2167702617747074.

"Anxiety and Phobias." Anxiety.org. Accessed October 2020. anxiety.org/phobias.

"Anxiety." Anxiety Care UK. Accessed October 2020. anxietycare.org.uk/anxiety.

Arch, Joanna J., and Michelle G. Craske. "First-line treatment: A critical appraisal of cognitive behavioral therapy developments and alternatives." *The Psychiatric Clinics of North America* 32, no. 3 (September 2009): 525–547. doi:10.1016/j.psc.2009.05.001.

Barlow, D. H. *Anxiety and Its Disorders. The Nature and Treatment of Anxiety and Panic*. 2nd ed. New York: Guilford Press, 2004.

Barlow, D. H. *The Clinical Handbook of Physiological Disorders*. 5th ed. New York: Guilford Press, 2014.

Barnett, Lauren A., Mark G. Pritchard, John J. Edwards, Ebenezer K. Afolabi, Kelvin P. Jordan, Emma L. Healey, Andrew G. Finney, Carolyn A. Chew-Graham, Christian D. Mallen, and Krysia S. Dziedzic. "Relationship of anxiety with joint pain and its management: A population survey." *Musculoskeletal Care* 16, no. 3 (September 2018): 353–362. doi:10.1002/msc.1243.

Beck, J. S. *Cognitive Behavior Therapy. Basics and Beyond*. 2nd ed. New York: Guilford Press, 2011.

Bokma, Wicher A., Neeltje M. Batelaan, Anton J. L. M. van Balkom, and Brenda W. J. H. Penninx. "Impact of anxiety and/or depressive disorders and chronic somatic diseases on disability and work impairment." *Journal of Psychosomatic Research* 94 (2017): 10–16. doi:10.1016/j.jpsychores.2017.01.004.

Brown, Kirk W., and Richard M. Ryan. "The benefits of being present: The role of mindfulness in psychological well-being." *Journal of Personality and Social Psychology* 84 (2003): 822–848.

Chapman, Robin A. *Integrating Clinical Hypnosis and CBT: Treating Depression, Anxiety, and Fears.* New York: Springer Publishing Company, 2014.

Clark, D. A., and Beck, A. T. *The Anxiety & Worry Workbook; The Cognitive Behavioral Solution.* New York: Guilford Press, 2012.

"Cognitive behavioral therapy." Institute for Quality and Efficiency in Health Care. September 8, 2016. ncbi.nlm.nih.gov/books/NBK279297.

Cox, Brian J., Richard P. Swinson, Ian D. Shulman, Klaus Kuch, and Jaak T. Reichman. "Gender effects and alcohol use in panic disorder with agoraphobia." *Behaviour Research and Therapy* 31, no. 4 (May 1993): 413–416.

D'Argembeau, Arnaud, Olivier Renaud, and Martial Van der Linden. "Frequency, characteristics and functions of future-oriented thoughts in daily life." *Applied Cognitive Psychology* 25 no. 1 (January 2011): 96–103. doi:10.1002/acp.1647.

Diagnostic and Statistical Manual of Mental Health Disorders, Fifth Edition. Arlington: American Psychiatric Publishing, 2013.

"The diathesis-stress model." APA Dictionary of Psychology. Accessed October 2020. dictionary.apa.org/diathesis-stress-model.

Dobson, Deborah, and Keith Dobson. "Avoidance in the clinic: Strategies to conceptualize and reduce avoidant thoughts, emotions, and behaviors with cognitive-behavioral therapy." *Practice Innovations* 3, no. 1 (January 2018): 32–42. doi.10.1037/pri0000061.

Doyle, Arthur C. *A Study in Scarlet.* United Kingdom: Ward Locke & Co., 1887.

Eifert, Georg H., and John P. Forsyth. *Acceptance and Commitment Therapy for Anxiety Disorders: A Practitioner's Treatment Guide to Using Mindfulness, Acceptance, and Values-Based Behavior Change Strategies.* Oakland: New Harbinger Publications, 2006.

Esfahani Smith, Emily. "There's more to life than being happy." April 2017. Video, 12:10. ted.com/talks/emily_esfahani_smith_there_s_more_to_life_than_being_happy.

Fernie, Bruce A., Zinnia Bharucha, Ana Nikčević, Claudia Marino, and Marcantonio Spada. "A metacognitive model of procrastination." *Journal of Affective Disorders* 210 (March 2017), 196–203. doi:10.1016/j.jad.2016.12.042.

Frank, Dana L., Lamees Khorshid, Jerome F. Kiffer, Moravec, C. S., & McKee, M. G. "Biofeedback in Medicine: Who, when, why and how?" *Mental Health in Family Medicine* 7, no. 2, 85–91.

Galinsky, Ellen, Kerstin Aumann, and James T. Bond. "Times are Changing: Gender and Generation at Work and at Home in the USA." *Expanding the Boundaries of Work-Family Research* 2013: 279–296. doi:10.1057/9781137006004_13.

Gayde, Levi. "What part of the brain deals with anxiety? What can brains affected by anxiety tell us?" BrainFacts.org. June 29, 2018. brainfacts.org/diseases-and-disorders/mental-health /2018/what-part-of-the-brain-deals-with-anxiety-what-can-brains-affected-by-anxiety-tell -us-062918.

"General information on clinical hypnosis." American Society of Clinical Hypnosis. Accessed October 2020. asch.net/Public/GeneralInfoonHypnosis/GeneralInfoTemplate.aspx.

Gottschalk, Michael G., and Katharina Domschke. (2017). "Genetics of generalized anxiety disorder and related traits." *Dialogues in Clinical Neuroscience* 19, no. 2 (June 2017): 159–168.

Grupe, Dan W., and Nitschke, Jack B. "Uncertainty and anticipation in anxiety: an integrated neurobiological and psychological perspective." *Nature Reviews Neuroscience* 14 (June 2013): 488–501. doi:10.1038/nrn3524.

Hadlandsmyth, Katherine, Diane L. Rosenbaum, Jennifer M. Craft, Ernest V. Gervino, and Kamila S. White. "Health care utilization in patients with non-cardiac chest pain: A longitudinal analysis of chest pain, anxiety and interoceptive fear." *Psychology & Health* 28, no. 8 (August 2013): 849–861. doi:10.1080/08870446.2012.762100.

Harding, Edward C., Nicholas P. Franks, and William Wisden. "Sleep and thermoregulation." *Current Opinion in Physiology* 15 (June 2020): 7–13. doi:10.1016/j.cophys .2019.11.008.

Harris, N., J. Baker, and R. Gray, eds. *Medicines Management in Mental Health Care.* West Sussex: Blackwell, 2009.

Harris, Russell. "Embracing your demons: An overview of acceptance and commitment therapy." Psychotherapy.net. Accessed October 2020. psychotherapy.net/article /Acceptance-and-Commitment-Therapy-ACT.

Hirsch, Collette, and Andrew Mathews. "A cognitive model of pathological worry." *Behaviour Research and Therapy* 50, no. 10 (October 2012): 636–646. doi:10.1016 /j.brat.2012.06.007.

Hofmann, Stefan G., and Aleena Hay. "Rethinking avoidance: Toward a balanced approach to avoidance in treating anxiety disorders." *Journal of Anxiety Disorders* 55 (April 2018): 14–21.

Hofmann, Stefan G., Anu Asnaani, Imke J. J. Vonk, Alice T. Sawyer, and Angela Fang. "The efficacy of cognitive behavioral therapy: A review of meta-analyses." *Cognitive Therapy and Research* 36, no. 5 (October 2012): 427–440. doi:10.1007/s10608-012-9476.

Im, Hwi-Jin, Yoon-Jung Kim, Hyeong-Geug Kim, Hyo-Seon Kim, and Chang-Gue Son. "Kouksundo, a traditional Korean mind-body practice, regulates oxidative stress profiles and stress hormones." *Physiology & Behavior* 141 (March 2015): 9–16. doi:10.1016/j.physbeh.2014.12.049.

"Impact of anxiety and depression on student academic progress." International Board of Credentialing and Continuing Education Standards. May 1, 2019. ibcces.org/blog/2019/05/01/impact-anxiety-depression-student-progress.

Kaczkurkin, Antonia N., and Edna B. Foa. "Cognitive-behavioral therapy for anxiety disorders: an update on the empirical evidence." *Dialogues in Clinical Neuroscience* 17, no. 3 (September 2015): 337–346. doi:10.31887/DCNS.2015.17.3/akaczkurkin.

Kirillov, Andrey Vladimirovich, Dina Tanatova Kabdullinova, Mikhail Vasilievich Vinichenko, and Sergey Anatolyevich Makushkin. "Theory and practice of time-management in education." *Asian Social Science* 11, no. 19 (July 2015): 193–204. doi:10.5539/ass.v11n19p193.

Komada, Yoko, Aoki Kazuyuki, Seiichi Gohshi, and Hideki Ichioka. "Effects of television luminance and wavelength at habitual bedtime on melatonin and cortisol secretion in humans: Blue light and melatonin secretion." *Sleep and Biological Rhythms* 13, no. 4 (May 2015): 316–322. doi:10.1111/sbr.12121.

Krypotos, Angelos-Miltiadis, Marieke Effting., Merel Kindt., and Tom Beckers. "Avoidance learning: a review of theoretical models and recent developments." *Behavioral Neuroscience* 9 (2015): 189.

Ladouceur, Robert, Michel J. Dugas, Mark Freeston, Eliane Léger, Fabien Gagnon, and Nicole Thibodeau. "Efficacy of a cognitive–behavioral treatment for generalized anxiety disorder: Evaluation in a controlled clinical trial." *Journal of Consulting and Clinical Psychology* 68, no. 6 (January 2001): 957–964. doi:10.1037/0022-006X.68.6.957.

Lissek, Shmuel. "Toward an account of clinical anxiety predicated on basic, neurally mapped mechanisms of Pavlovian fear-learning: The case for conditioned overgeneralization." *Depression and Anxiety* 29, no. 4 (April 2012): 257–263. doi:10.1002/da.21922.

Lissek, Shmuel, Stephanie Rabin, Randi E. Heller, David Lukenbaugh, Marilla Geraci, Daniel S. Pine, and Christian Grillon. (2010). "Overgeneralization of conditioned fear as a pathogenic marker of panic disorder." *American Journal of Psychiatry* 167, no. 1 (January 2010): 47–55. doi:10.1176/appi.ajp.2009.09030410.

Longe, J. *The Gale Encyclopedia of Psychology*. Farmington Hills: Cengage Gale, 2016.

McLean, Carmen P., Anu Asnaani, Brett T. Litz, and Stefan G. Hofmann. "Gender differences in anxiety disorders: prevalence, course of illness, comorbidity and burden of illness." *Journal of Psychiatric Research* 45, no. 8 (August 2011): 1027–1035. doi:10.1016/j.jpsychires.2011.03.006.

Measuring Wellbeing: A Guide for Practitioners. London: New Economics Foundation, 2012. b.3cdn.net/nefoundation/8d92cf44e70b3d16e6_rgm6bpd3i.pdf.

"Meditation: In Depth." National Center for Complementary and Integrative Health. April 2016. nccih.nih.gov/health/meditation-in-depth.

Meek, William. "Generalized anxiety disorder: Causes and risk factors." VeryWellMind. July 10, 2020. verywellmind.com/gad-causes-risk-factors-1392982.

Miller, W., and S. Rollnick. *Motivational Interviewing: Helping People Change*. 3rd ed. New York: Guilford Press, 2013.

Morris, Laura O. "Dizziness related to anxiety and stress." Vestibular Rehabilitation. August 2015. neuropt.org/docs/default-source/vsig-english-pt-fact-sheets/anxiety-and-stress-dizziness4ca035a5390366a68a96ff00001fc240.pdf?sfvrsn=80a35343_0&sfvrsn=80a35343_0.

Neudeck, Peter, and Hans-Ulrich Wittchen, eds. *Exposure Therapy: Rethinking the Model, Refining the Method*. New York: Springer Publishing, 2012.

Nightingale, Earl. *The Strangest Secret*. Recorded 1966. Nightingale-McHugh Company. Vinyl.

Norton, Alice R., and Maree J. Abbott. "The Role of Environmental Factors in the Aetiology of Social Anxiety Disorder: A Review of the Theoretical and Empirical Literature." *Behaviour Change* 34, no. 2 (May 2017): 76–97. doi:10.1017/bec.2017.7.

N, Pam. "Avoidance." PsychologyDictionary.org. April 7, 2013. psychologydictionary.org/avoidance.

Nutt, David J., and James C. Ballenger, eds. *Anxiety Disorders*. Wiley-Blackwell, 2008.

Ochoa, Lourdes, Aaron T. Beck, and Robert A. Steer. "Gender differences in comorbid anxiety and mood disorders." *American Journal of Psychiatry* 149, no. 10 (1992): 1409–1410. doi:10.1176/ajp.149.10.1409b.

O'Leary, Ann. "Stress, emotion, and human immune function." *Psychological Bulletin* 108, no. 3 (1990): 363–382. doi:10.1037/0033-2909.108.3.363.

Osherson, Samuel, and Steven Krugman. "Men, shame, and psychotherapy." *Psychotherapy: Theory, Research, Practice, Training* 27, no. 3 (Fall 1990): 327–339. doi:10.1037/0033-3204.27.3.327.

Oshio, Atsushi. "Development and validation of the dichotomous thinking inventory." *Social Behavior and Personality* 37, no. 6 (July 2009): 729–741. doi:10.2224/sbp .2009.37.6.729.

Otte, Christian. "Cognitive behavioral therapy in anxiety disorders: Current state of the evidence." *Dialogues in Clinical Neuroscience* 13, no. 4 (December 2011): 413–421.

"Panic attacks and panic disorder." Mayo Clinic. May 4, 2018. mayoclinic.org/diseases -conditions/panic-attacks/symptoms-causes/syc-20376021.

Parker, Gordon Barraclough, and Heather Lorraine Brotchie. "From diathesis to dimorphism: The biology of gender differences in depression." *The Journal of Nervous and Mental Disease* 192, no. 3 (March 2004): 210–216. doi: 10.1097/01.nmd.0000116464.60500.63.

Pelletier, Kenneth R. "Mind-body health: research, clinical, and policy applications." *American Journal of Health Promotion* 6, no. 5 (May 1992): 345–358. doi:10.4278 /0890-1171-6.5.345.

Ramis, Harold, dir. *Groundhog Day*. United States: Columbia Pictures, 1993. 101 minutes.

"Results from the 2010 National Survey on Drug Use and Health: Mental Health Findings." US Department of Health and Human Services. New York: Aspen Publishers, 2011.

Rosqvist, Johan. *Exposure Treatments for Anxiety Disorders: A Practitioner's Guide to Concepts, Methods, and Evidence-Based Practice*. New York: Taylor & Francis Group, 2005.

Schechter, Nevit. "How to stop a panic attack: triggers, signs and coping strategies." NetDoctor. May 11, 2020. netdoctor.co.uk/healthy-living/mental-health/a27053543 /panic-attack-treatment.

Schmidt, A; Thews, G. "Autonomic nervous system." In Janig, W. (ed.) *Human Physiology*. 2nd ed. New York: Springer-Verlag, 1989. 333–370. doi:10.1007/978-3-642-96211-0_8.

Seif, Martin N., and Sally Winston. *What Every Therapist Needs to Know About Anxiety Disorders: Key Concepts, Insights and Interventions*. New York: Routledge, 2014.

Simos, Gregoris, and Stefan G. Hofmann. *CBT for Anxiety Disorders: A Practitioner Book*. West Sussex: John Wiley & Sons, 2013.

Steimer, Thierry. "The biology of fear and anxiety-related behaviors." *Dialogues in Clinical Neuroscience* 4, no. 3 (September 2002): 231–249. 10.31887/DCNS.2002.4.3/tsteimer.

Tiger, Lionel. *Men in Groups*. New York: Routledge, 2017.

Tompkins, Michael A. *Anxiety and Avoidance: A Universal Treatment for Anxiety, Panic, and Fear*. Oakland: New Harbinger Publications, 2013.

Toohey, Michael J. "Irritability characteristics and parameters in an international sample." *Journal of Affective Disorders* 263 (February 2020): 558–567. doi:10.1016/j.jad.2019.11.021.

Watkins, Ed, Michelle Moulds, and Bundy Mackintosh. "Comparisons between rumination and worry in a non-clinical population." *Behaviour Research and Therapy* 43, no. 12:1577–1585. doi:10.1016/j.brat.2004.11.008.

Westbrook, David, Helen Kennerley, and Joan Kirk. *An Introduction to Cognitive Behaviour Therapy: Skills and applications*. 2nd ed. Sage: 2011.

"What is exposure therapy?" American Psychological Association. July 2017. apa.org/ptsd-guideline/patients-and-families/exposure-therapy.

"World health statistics 2018: Monitoring health for the SDGs, sustainable development goals." World Health Organization. May 21, 2019. who.int/publications/i/item/world-health-statistics-2019-monitoring-health-for-the-sdgs-sustainable-development-goals.

Zemeckis, Robert, dir. *Back to the Future*. United States: Universal Pictures, 1985. 116 minutes.

Zinbarg, Richard E., Michelle G. Craske, and David H. Barlow. *Mastery of Your Anxiety and Worry: Therapist Guide*. 2nd ed. New York: Oxford University Press, 2006.

Index

A

Acceptance, 45, 76-77, 91-94
Acceptance and commitment
    therapy (ACT), 45
Accountability partners, 109-110
Adverse childhood experiences (ACEs), 12
Affirmations, 62
Ambiguity. *See* Uncertainty
American Psychiatric Association, 15
Amygdala, 10
Anger, 6-7
Anxiety
  about, 9-11
  benefits of, 11
  and comorbid disorders, 5-7
  compensatory behaviors, 2-3
  expressions of, 2
  factors contributing to, 12
  vs. fear, 13
  forms of, 14-16
  in men vs. women, 2
  overcoming, 20, 166-171
  reluctance to seek help for, 2-5
Anxiety index, 17-19
Autonomic nervous system, 10
Autopilot mode, 133-134
Avoidance, 88-90. *See also* Procrastination
Awareness, 45, 132-134

B

Behavioral symptoms, 33-34
Biofeedback, 46
Body
  awareness, 132-134
  mind-body connection, 131
  physical symptoms, 9-10, 126-130

Brain, anxiety and, 10
Breathing exercises, 121, 152-153

C

CALM acronym, 34-35
Career, as a trigger, 25, 73
Chronotypes, 109
Clinical hypnotherapy, 46
Cognitive behavioral therapy (CBT), 42-44
Cognitive distortions
  dichotomous thinking, 52-55
  jumping to conclusions, 58-60
  overgeneralizing, 55-57
Cognitive errors, 52
Cognitive restructuring, 60-68
Cognitive symptoms, 32-33
Comorbid disorders, 5-7
Competition, 75
Confirmation bias, 58
Conflict, 75
Coping behaviors
  acceptance, 91-94
  active coping, 95
  avoidance, 88-90
  substance abuse, 6, 97
Co-vitality, 25
Critical thinking, 65-67
Cultural norms, 3-4

D

Daily life, as a trigger, 25-26
Default mode network (DMN), 132-133
Depression, 7
Desensitization, 138-140, 142
Detachment, 67

Diagnostic and Statistical Manual of Mental Health Disorders, Fifth Edition (DSM-5), 9, 14

Diaphragmatic breathing, 152–153

Diet and nutrition, 158–159

E

Education, as a trigger, 25

Emotional suppression, 5, 96–97

Emotions
acceptance of, 92–93
engaging with, 96–97
overwhelming, 95
sharing, 98

Engagement coping, 88

Environmental factors, 12

Exercise, 159

Exposure therapy
about, 45–46, 94–95
desensitization, 138–140, 142
gradual vs. flooding, 138
habituation, 140
interoceptive, 139
obstacles to, 146–147
safely practicing, 141
in vivo vs. imaginal, 138–139

F

Failure, fear of, 102–104

Fear. *See also* Exposure therapy
vs. anxiety, 13
facing, 142–145
of failure, 102–104
hierarchy, 139
network, 10

Fight-or-flight response, 10, 31

Financial situations, 74

G

Generalized anxiety disorder (GAD), 14–15, 34

Genetic factors, 12

Goal-setting, 36–38

Growth, 166–170

Guided imagery, 154–155

H

Habituation, 140

Health, as a trigger, 25, 74

Hypnosis, 46

I

Insecurity, 3

Irritability, 7

J

Jacobson, Edmund, 152

Journaling, 156

M

Mantras, 99

Maslow, Abraham, 10

Medications, 160

Meditation, 45, 120

Mental health support
emergency, 11
reluctance to seek, 2–5
treatment approaches, 42–46

Mind-body connection, 131

Mindfulness practices, 45
body awareness, 132–134
for worry, 115–117

N

National Suicide Prevention Lifeline, 11

P

Panic attacks, 16, 31, 34, 117–122

"Paper tigers," 13, 116

Parasympathetic nervous system, 10

Phobias, 15, 34

Physical symptoms, 9–10, 31–32, 126–130

Procrastination, 102–111

Progressive muscle relaxation
(PMR), 121, 153–154
Progressive Relaxation (Jacobson), 152

R

Radical acceptance, 76
Relationships, 74
Relaxation therapy, 152–155
Riptide visualization, 82
Rumination, 16

S

Self-actualization, 10
Self-care, 157–159, 169
Self-fulfilling prophecies, 63
Self-harm, 11
Sleep, 157–158
SMART analogy, 38
Smith, Emily Esfahani, 79
Social anxiety disorder (SAD), 15, 32–33, 34
Social interactions, 24–25, 73
Stigmas, mental health, 3–4
Substance abuse, 6, 97
Suicidal thoughts, 11
Support systems, 109–110, 170–171
Sympathetic nervous system, 10
Symptoms
behavioral, 33–34
cognitive, 32–33
panic attacks, 118–119
physical, 9–10, 31–32, 126–130

T

Thoughts and thinking
absolute, 54
automatic, 52

catastrophizing, 54
dichotomous, 54
expressing, 116
jumping to conclusions, 58–60
negative cycles, 52–53
overgeneralizing, 55–57
restructuring, 60–68
Treatment approaches
acceptance and commitment
therapy (ACT), 45
biofeedback, 46
clinical hypnotherapy, 46
cognitive behavioral therapy (CBT), 42–44
exposure therapy, 45–46, 94–95, 138–147
medications, 160
meditation, 45
mindfulness, 45
Triggers, 24–30, 113

U

Uncertainty
accepting, 76–80
causes of, 73–75
embracing, 80–82
responding to, 72–73
Unconditional self-acceptance, 76

V

Visualization, 82, 154–155

W

Well-being, 25
Worry, 16, 111–117
Worry time, 68

Acknowledgments

I want to offer an enormous thank-you to all my Kiwi, Aussie, Texan, and UK mates and colleagues who, over the years, have provided such incredible support and encouragement. With y'all in my corner, I have been able to find my voice.

I would like to acknowledge all the gentlemen who have found the courage to seek help and engage in conversation over the years. Therapy is a two-way street, and I continue to learn from you. I genuinely believe that the more that men talk, the better this world can be.

I especially want to thank my sons, Liam and Oscar, for being the inspiration for all I do and for all the joy and laughter you bring into my life. Keep seeking all the beauty and opportunity that life has to offer, my beautiful lads. *Kia Kaha*—stay strong!

This book wouldn't have been possible without the strength of the women in my life. To my mum, Barbara, the kindness in your heart is bigger than the sun. To my stepmum, Pauline, your sense of adventure and feistiness is infectious, and to my mother-in-law, Eva, your energy is addictive.

And most of all, I am humbled and extremely grateful to the rock in my life, my darling wife, Janene. Your strength, encouragement, and love are beyond measure. *Arohanui*, my sweet. This book would not have happened without you.

About the Author

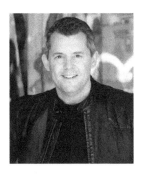

Simon G. Niblock, MA, LMFT, is a licensed marriage and family therapist in private practice in Austin, Texas, who specializes in tailored psychotherapy services for men.

Simon was born and raised free-range in New Zealand. He has lived and worked in Australia, Asia, Europe, the United Kingdom, and the United States, and he migrated into the practice of clinical psychotherapy after an extensive career in the high-tech software world. He has received formal training and education in Sydney, Australia, and Austin.

His greatest lessons in life have come from the humbling yet privileged roles of being an adoring husband and a father of two amazing sons.

For more information about Simon and the various services he provides, visit SimonNiblock.com.